DISASTER HANDBOOK

DISASTER HANDBOOK

SOLOMON GARB, M. D.

Associate Professor of Pharmacology,
School of Medicine, University of Missouri

EVELYN ENG, R. N., M. A.

Director of Nursing Service,
University Hospital, Columbia, Missouri

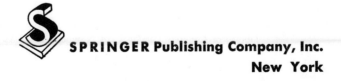

SPRINGER Publishing Company, Inc.
New York

PREFACE

This book has been planned primarily for doctors and nurses but we think that others interested in disaster casualty prevention and disaster management will also find it helpful. Since studies of major disasters have shown that most of the deaths and injuries—perhaps 95% of them—could have been prevented, we have emphasized prevention and outlined a number of preventive measures to avert casualties. But we also realize that it will be some time before all these measures can be put into effect and have, therefore, devoted an equal amount of space to describing ways and means of helping future disaster victims.

One fact that is illustrated by many disasters is that the effectiveness of individuals or groups depends not only on how well they do their own jobs but also on how well they allow others to do theirs. In other words, persons who might be called upon to render disaster aid should have a clear understanding of the capabilities and roles of other individuals and groups in disaster work; to facilitate such understanding we have outlined several ways in which persons or groups can be most helpful.

Studies of disaster and disaster management have certain disadvantages compared to studies of other phenomena and experiences. Trained observers are seldom present during the early phases of a disaster so that much of what we know is based on reconstruction of past events. In addition, there has been little, if any, opportunity to test new methods of handling the problems of disaster, so that suggestions for improvement are based on past experience instead of on controlled studies. Some of the suggestions contained in this book were originally made by others, some are the result of our own deductions and evaluations. Generally speaking, we have stressed basic concepts and have tried to give them substance, dimension and reality by providing detailed descriptions of a number of disasters.

The coverage of the various kinds of disaster differs. Our criterion has been the probable degree of the reader's involvement. For example, the persons for whom the *Handbook* is written can do a great deal to reduce the toll of fires. By contrast, mine disasters involve problems of such technical nature that few people are equipped to handle them, except in indirect ways; such disasters, therefore, are presented in less detail.

Our study of past disasters has convinced us that disaster must be dealt with as a phenomenon in its own right. Experience and training in non-disaster situations do not ordinarily qualify a person to take a position of leadership in a disaster—an observation that has been made by many who have studied disasters. We hope, therefore, that the information presented in the *Disaster Handbook* will help prepare more people to assume useful roles in the prevention and reduction of disaster casualties and in the caring for the victims.

We wish to express our gratitude to Henry M. Parrish, M.D., Dr.P.H., for writing the chapter on epidemiologic and public health aspects of disasters, and to Mrs. Joyce Pharriss for her efficient secretarial help.

SOLOMON GARB, M.D.
EVELYN ENG, R.N., M.A.

June 15, 1964
Columbia, Missouri

CONTENTS

chapter

1 INTRODUCTION

A disaster is a great, sudden misfortune resulting in loss of life, serious injury, and property loss. Strictly speaking, if such misfortune befalls even one person, it is a disaster. However, in current usage, the term is used to refer to a sudden occurrence which kills and injures relatively large numbers of persons. This is the sense in which the word "disaster" is used in this book. To be more specific, we will use the term to refer to a sudden occurrence which results in death or serious injury to 25 or more persons.

The toll of disasters is seldom fully realized by most persons. In the United States, approximately 1,300 people have died in disasters every year of this century. The number injured is about 13,000 to 15,000 per year. These figures apply only to the disasters killing 25 or more persons at a time. Many more people die each year in equivalent occurrences which take less than 25 lives. For example, about 10,000 die each year in small fires. However, even this does not tell the entire story. We have so far been spared from the really tremendous disasters. In some countries, a single disaster has killed as many people as we have lost in half a century. Disasters, then, constitute a serious problem, not only in individual but also in public health terms. Furthermore, studies of past disasters show that most deaths and injuries are preventable.

Part of the tragedy of many disasters is the fact that all or most of the casualties could have been prevented by relatively simple means. Often, there were several possible preventive measures that could have been taken anywhere along the sequence of events leading to the disaster, and any *one* of those preventive measures could have saved most of the lives lost. Let's consider some examples:

A. *The Texas City fire and explosion of 1947—561 deaths.* Any *one* of the following would have prevented or minimized the casualties:

1. Realization by the crew of the Grandcamp that ammonium nitrate doesn't need oxygen to burn, that an ammonium nitrate fire cannot be extinguished by steam, and that only large amounts of cold water could extinguish the fire.

2. Reporting the fire by radio to the United States Coast Guard at once, with request for advice and guidance.

1

3. Evacuation of the area near the fire by police.

4. Restraint of curious sightseers who came to the dock to watch.

B. *The Chicago school fire of 1958—95 deaths.* Any *one* of the following would have prevented all or most of the deaths:

1. Proper design of the school, with adequate exits.

2. Installation of an automatic sprinkler system.

3. Good housekeeping, preventing accumulation of combustible trash.

4. Immediate sounding of the fire alarm as soon as smoke was smelled.

5. Immediate notification of the city fire department as soon as smoke was smelled.

C. *The sinking of the Titanic—1,517 deaths.* Any *one* of the following would have prevented all or most of the deaths:

1. Steering a more prudent course, out of range of icebergs.

2. Heeding iceberg warnings given by passing ships.

3. Safe speeds, without attempts to set a record.

4. Provision of enough lifeboats.

5. Proper lifeboat drills.

It may be noted that although some of these precautions are now in general use, all are still not universally employed. In 1959, another ship —the Hans Hedtoft—collided with an iceberg in almost the same fashion as the Titanic, and 95 lives were lost.

These examples can be extended with many others. In approaching the problems of disasters, therefore, prevention will be emphasized. Prevention has several facets. Prevention of the disaster itself is feasible in certain types, such as fires, explosions, and collapse of buildings. In most cases, even if prevention of the initial occurrence (such as earthquake, hurricane, tornado) is impossible, prevention or reduction of loss of lives is quite possible. An excellent example of this point is provided by some hurricane statistics. Two hurricanes struck the same area four years apart. The first killed 430 people, the second, a more severe storm, killed 40. The difference was the result of soundly planned, effectively executed disaster control plans. Finally, preventive measures can be of great value in saving lives from secondary effects of a disaster—a phase which has not yet received the attention its importance deserves.

Studies of past disasters have called attention to the disorganization of the efforts to provide help. In some cases, the disorganization caused needless extra casualties; in all cases, it prevented the carrying out of optimum life-saving measures. Accordingly, this book will emphasize the value of organization—including organization of our knowledge and understanding of the phenomena involved, and organization of the efforts to prevent casualties and help the injured.

The importance of learning about disasters, and of training people in the appropriate techniques of dealing with them also must be considered. It would be a serious error to assume that a person, even though professionally trained in a related field, would necessarily function effectively in a disaster without further instruction and training. To be sure, many persons without such training have been able to adjust rapidly enough to the disorder and confusion of the disaster scene to do an excellent job. However, they probably would have done an even better job if they had known more about disasters. Furthermore, there is convincing evidence that in several disasters, even doctors—including highly trained surgeons—were so caught up in the disorder and confusion as to be unable to function effectively. Every person, therefore, who may be involved in a disaster should learn as much as possible about disasters, as well as about their prevention and their management.

BASIC FEATURES OF DISASTERS

This section contains some of the basic features of disasters and of disaster management, considered in general terms; in addition, it presents some of the problems which have arisen in the past and their possible solutions.

2 THE MISSION

The mission of disaster management is basically the prevention and minimization of death, disability, suffering, and loss. The methods of carrying out this mission will vary with the type of disaster, its location, and the professional background of the individual. Thus, the doctor and nurse are likely to concentrate on different aspects than the policeman, fireman, or civil defense volunteer. However, there are certain fundamental principles which should be thoroughly understood by *everyone* who may have a responsibility for helping the victims of a disaster. Furthermore, it is important that these principles be applied in the proper sequence, lest they lose effectiveness or cause even more deaths and injuries.

There are eight basic principles, and it is recommended that they be thoroughly memorized in the proper sequence:

1. *Prevent* the occurrence of the disaster, whenever possible.
2. *Minimize the number of casualties* if the disaster cannot be prevented.
3. *Prevent further casualties* from occurring after the initial impact of the disaster.
4. *Rescue the victims.*
5. *Provide first aid* to the injured.
6. *Evacuate the injured* to medical installations.
7. *Provide definitive medical care.*
8. *Promote the reconstruction* of the lives of victims.

Let us illustrate the importance of this listing with some examples from past disasters, and show how past experiences suggest the need for more knowledge of and training in these areas. (In subsequent chapters we will try to show how these principles apply to each disaster under consideration.)

Prevention of disaster is practical for certain types of disasters, but not as yet for others. The preventable disasters may be divided into those which actually are being prevented, and those which are partially or inadequately prevented. For example, we have prevented epidemics of smallpox, cholera, typhoid and diphtheria by means of vaccination and good public health measures. Some fires have been prevented by enforcement of good building codes; some floods have been prevented or modified by proper soil management and dam construction. As we consider each type of disaster in a systematic fashion, asking "Could this have been prevented?," we will note that the answer for many is "yes." Unfortunately, however, the professions which are largely concerned with disaster management are not yet exerting their full influence in bringing about adequate preventive measures. One of the major aims of this book is the development of a disaster-prevention attitude. In the past, it has taken one or more dramatic disasters to arouse the public to the need for adequate preventive measures. Sometimes, even a dramatic disaster has not been enough to stimulate thorough, nationwide preventive measures. In the Red Cross publication *Disaster,* this question was asked: "Must we wait for a major disaster like the Collinwood, Ohio school fire with its 175 youthful victims before we investigate fire safety conditions in our schools?"* Unfortunately, the Collinwood fire in 1908 was not— apparently—enough of a stimulus to make schools safe from fire. In 1958, a school in Chicago burned, killing 95 persons and injuring many more. A year later, 24 were killed in a school fire near Little Rock, Arkansas. Hospitals and nursing homes seem to be particularly susceptible to disastrous fires. In 1949, 77 people died in a hospital fire in Illinois; a year later, 41 died in an Iowa hospital fire; in 1953, 35 died in a Florida nursing home fire; four years later, 72 perished in a Missouri home for the aged, and in 1961, 16 lost their lives in the Hartford, Connecticut, fire. All these disasters were preventable. Clearly, *disaster prevention* has been insufficient in these areas, despite the presence of educated, intelligent professional personnel right on the scene.

The second basic principle—*minimizing the number of casualties if the disaster cannot be prevented*—is now being effectively applied in hurricanes. We don't know how to prevent hurricanes, but through proper education, training, and warning, we have been able to reduce deaths and injuries by a large margin. Before these measures were taken hurricanes were among the most serious disasters to strike the United States. In 1957, hurricane "Audrey" killed 430 in Texas and Louisiana. Vigorous measures were taken to prevent such casualties in future storms. A few years later, hurricane "Carla"—even more powerful than "Audrey" —struck the same area, and, as mentioned before, only 40 died.

The third principle—*preventing further casualties after initial impact* —may at first seem a minor modification of the second principle. However, it involves types of action quite different from those in other meas-

* *Disaster, I:* 3, 1947.

ures, and therefore deserves separate consideration. Furthermore, this principle has been widely overlooked in past disasters and as a result many lives were lost that could have easily been saved.

The impact of many disasters is followed by an unstable situation in which a number of events, dangerous to life, may occur. For example, after many disasters secondary fires break out which sometimes do more damage than the original disaster, as was the case in the San Francisco earthquake.

It is easy to understand why untrained people usually ignore or are unaware of this principle. A disaster strikes—they run to aid the victims or to look at the spectacle. Without special training, they are not likely to stop, look and ask: "Can any other danger be in the offing?"

A secondary disaster of great magnitude was prevented after the Worcester tornado because well-trained professional firemen automatically applied the proper principle. The first Worcester firemen arrived on the scene within a few minutes after the tornado had passed. They saw the dead and the injured; they also saw piles of inflammable lumber from destroyed homes and at least six fires just starting. The firemen did not rush to give first aid to the victims—instead, they put the fires out and kept them out. A subsequent study showed that this action probably prevented a conflagration which would have killed many more people than had the tornado.

Prevention of further casualties from secondary effects of a disaster, therefore, should ordinarily take precedence over first aid and evacuation of the injured. Every person in a position of responsibility at a disaster scene should ask himself, "Is there any likelihood of a secondary disaster?" *before* starting with first-aid measures. If there is a likelihood of a secondary disaster, steps to prevent or minimize it should be undertaken at once. Furthermore, even if the scene seems safe at first, *continuous* checks of the area are needed to provide adequate protection. A sound procedure is to designate a responsible person as a safety officer, with the sole duty of watching the scene and sounding a warning in case of an impending secondary disaster.

The fourth principle—*rescue*—includes the locating and freeing of persons trapped in debris, and bringing flood victims to higher ground. Competent, trained rescue teams will usually save many more lives than untrained volunteers with inadequate leadership and direction. According to one authority, commenting on a tornado disaster, "many died who might have lived had there been an effective rescue and evacuation team. In fact, as I saw the earlier evacuation efforts, it is miraculous that more did not die. I saw many school boys as well as grown men chopping and sawing at beams, which held up whole sections of roof and tons of bricks, in ignorant and feeble rescue attempts."* In rescue, as in other measures, vigorous action and good intentions are no substitutes for training and knowledge.

The fifth principle—*providing first aid to the injured*—has frequently been ignored in disasters, or has been inadequate. The average American, faced with a large number of casualties, apparently forgets or ignores whatever he has learned of first aid and tries to get the victim to the hospital as soon as possible. In past disasters, therefore, many patients have arrived at hospitals in shock, and with simple fractures changed into compound fractures. In almost all disasters which have been studied, attempts had been made to set up first-aid stations. However, these first-aid stations had largely been by-passed in the rush to the hospitals. In general, less than 10% of the victims arriving at the hospitals show evidence of having had first aid. It must be emphasized that first aid is not a substitute for definitive treatment, nor a stopgap until the patient sees a doctor. Instead, it is just what the name implies—the first step in aiding the patient; and unless the first step is undertaken promptly, subsequent treatments may be much less effective, or the patient may even die before these can be instituted.

The sixth step—*evacuating the injured to medical installations*—is usually done vigorously and rapidly but improperly. As pointed out above, the victims are usually transported without benefit of first aid, so that their injuries become more severe. The experience in the Worcester tornado showed that overemphasis on speed worsened the conditions of several victims who were driven at high speeds over rough roads. Nothing was gained by this speed because there was already a long line of injured at the hospital, awaiting treatment.

Included in proper evacuation procedures are measures to route the injured to hospitals in a balanced fashion. This has seldom been done in the past. Usually, the hospitals nearest to the scene are swamped with casualties, with the result that many patients have to wait hours, and even days, for definitive care, while hospitals a few miles away receive very few patients and have practically no casualties to care for.

The seventh principle—*providing definitive medical care*—also depends for its effectiveness on prior planning and training. The usual training of doctors and nurses, as well as the hospital plans, are seldom

* Hertel, J. Unpublished report quoted by Raker, J. W., et al. *Emergency Medical Care in Disasters.* Disaster Study Number 6. National Research Council Publication 457, Washington, D. C., 1956, p. 21.

enough for efficient handling of a large number of disaster victims. Under the pressures of large numbers of casualties, ordinary procedures break down. Surgeons, for instance, have become confused, have abandoned sound operative procedures and sutured contaminated wounds. One chief of surgery did not recognize the fact that his greatest contribution to the victims' would have been the supervision of surgery. Instead, he spent his time carrying litters, a job which many unskilled, untrained onlookers could have handled.

In many disasters, lack of planning or poor planning by hospital administrators has resulted in unnecessary delays in furnishing definitive care.

The final principle—*promoting the reconstruction of the lives of the victims*—begins as soon as the initial medical and surgical procedures are over. The way in which the disaster is discussed, and the opportunities the victims have to talk about their experiences, may have considerable bearing on their eventual adjustments. In this area, too, good intentions and energetic measures are not enough in themselves. Actual experiences and lessons of past disasters must be studied to find out which actions were helpful and which harmful.

3 CHRONOLOGY AND GEOGRAPHY OF DISASTER

The chronology of disaster is an artificial division of the time elements in a disaster situation. Since it is helpful to have uniformity in the terms used, we will use the outline developed by others. An understanding of the chronology is an important base for planning. The following phases are generally recognized in the literature on disaster: Threat → Warning → Impact → Inventory → Rescue → Remedy → Recovery.

The *threat phase* may be entirely absent, as in the case of an earthquake. However, in most disasters there is a definite threat phase which may last from minutes to weeks. Unfortunately, the threat is often unrecognized or minimized. Early recognition of the threat, though, is vital to the prevention of many disasters and the reduction of casualties in most others. Examples of threat phases are: 1) Heavy rains and melting snows which may present a threat of flooding. 2) Discovery of a hurricane far out at sea. 3) Identification of certain temperature and pressure relations in the air which are associated with tornadoes. 4) Excessive drought in a wooded area which may present a threat of forest fires. 5) Storage of highly inflammable materials in areas vulnerable to fire which may present a threat of a major fire. Most threats, however, fail to materialize into actual disasters.

The *warning phase* is usually much shorter, ranging from seconds to hours, and implies a very high probability that disaster may strike. (It may be non-existent in earthquakes.) There is usually no time to try to prevent the disaster, but there is often time enough to take shelter or to get away from the disaster area. Everyone should learn to recognize the warning phase. Some examples are:

1. The sighting of a funnel cloud denotes a tornado.
2. Information from the weather bureau that a hurricane course has been plotted and the storm will strike the coast in a short time.
3. A regression of the water level on the shores of the ocean is a warning of an impending tsunami (tidal wave).
4. Smoke over a dry forest is a warning of impending forest fire.
5. Reports of rising river levels are warnings of floods to come.

The *impact phase* is the time during which the disaster is actually present in the particular area. In earthquakes and explosions the impact

CHRONOLOGY AND GEOGRAPHY   13

phase may last less than a minute. In fires and floods the impact may last more than a day. It should be noted that not all the casualties are produced during the impact phase. Often, additional casualties are produced after the primary impact has passed, mainly because of the unstable situations that remain after the impact. Some refer to these situations as secondary impacts.

The *inventory phase,* which follows the impact, is one in which the victims, their neighbors, and the general community look around and take stock of what has happened, and determine what their situation is. There is no clear-cut transition from the inventory phase to the *rescue phase.* While one person is still looking around in a partial daze, another may have started to rescue his family and neighbors. The rescue phase also overlaps into the remedy phase.

The *remedy phase* includes the time when first aid is given, evacuation is accomplished, and definitive medical care obtained.

The *recovery phase* constitutes the time needed to return to a relatively stable and balanced way of life. It may last from weeks to years, depending on the type of disaster and the people involved.

The recovery phase is one which has received relatively little notice. It is undramatic and unspectacular. Many presentations of disaster show a picture of the devastation shortly after impact, together with a picture of the same area a year or two later. The second picture is of a flourishing, rebuilt community, often better looking than it had been originally. There is little doubt that the physical appearance of an area which has been rebuilt after a disaster is often superior to its predisaster situation. The natural impulse upon comparing the pictures is to assume that the physical reconstruction of the disaster area parallels the personal reconstruction of the lives of the people involved. Unfortunately, the few studies which have been done of this phase show that reconstruction of the lives of the victims proceeds more slowly and less satisfactorily than the physical reconstruction.

The geographic divisions of the total area concerned with a disaster were conceived in order to clarify the arising problems and help manage them. There are three major divisions: the impact area, the filter area, and the community-aid area.

The *impact area* is the one in which the disaster strikes, causing its casualties.

The *filter area* is the location around the impact area in which notification of the area is immediate and direct. That is, people in the filter area see or hear the disaster strike the impact area. The filter area usually surrounds the impact area completely, but its extent will vary with the type of disaster. In a crash, the filter area may be only a few hundred feet wide; in a major fire or explosion, it may be miles wide. The appropriateness of the word "filter" for this area can be judged best after reading chapter 9. In general, aid to the impact area starts to flow from the filter area immediately, without any need for notification.

The *community-aid area* is that additional area from which help flows to the impact area. Notification of the community-aid area is apt to be slow and highly selective.

4 PSYCHOLOGY OF DISASTER

The psychology of disaster involves several distinct facets. There is the psychology of the victim before, during, and after the disaster, of the volunteer helper, the trained professional, and the onlooker. Each should be understood in order to cope with the problems which he presents.

The Victim

Most people believe that a disaster is something that happens to someone else—not to themselves or their families. This is called the "delusion of personal invulnerability." As a result, they are likely to ignore or minimize warnings, and refrain from taking preventive measures. The delusion of personal invulnerability is in many ways comforting, and people don't like to give it up. At times, if they are pressed by authorities or by events themselves to take protective measures, they react with hostility. This is, of course, an immature attitude, but quite a common one. It is seen clearly in much of the opposition to civil defense. Many people just do not wish to face and consider the possibility of being killed or seriously injured, and become angry at those who ask that they do face these possibilities.

Therefore, responsible persons, trying to train and educate the general population in ways of protecting themselves against disaster, should expect to meet a substantial degree of indifference and hostility. Techniques must be developed to counteract these responses.

During the warning phase, the average person tends to picture the oncoming disaster in the most optimistic framework of his past experiences. For example, when the Dutch government warned of the impending floods of 1953, many people in the danger area assumed that the flood would be a minor one, similar to one which had occurred years before— *even though the warnings said that the expected flood would be severe.* Some families lifted all items off the floor and put them on chairs so they wouldn't get wet. As it happened, the floods covered their homes.

The delusion of personal invulnerability can be counteracted by vigorous training or by imaginative action or both. The city manager of Eagle Pass, Texas, used a simple but ingenious method to counter this delusion and get the residents of the city to evacuate to higher ground when news came of an impending flood of the Rio Grande. He painted a white line

on all the store windows in downtown Eagle Pass, showing the height
which the flood waters would reach in the streets. This, together with
other measures, convinced the residents that they should heed the warnings,
with the result that nobody died. The situation, however, was different
in the twin city of Piedras Negras, just across the river. Here, the residents refused to believe that a real disaster was threatening and ignored,
or even resisted, attempts to evacuate them. As a result, many died in
the flood.

Those persons who have ignored all warnings *before* the disaster
impact often overreact to warnings, rumors, and wild speculations *after* the
impact. This can cause serious problems in the impact and fringe areas.
The most effective and practical way of minimizing the harm from this
sort of psychologic pattern is the prompt setting up of an efficient communications system.

After the actual impact of the disaster, the attitude changes. There are
many popular misconceptions about responses in disaster. The major one
is the belief that panic is a frequent occurrence—actually, panic is quite
rare in most disasters and occurs only under certain specific circumstances.
Panic will be discussed separately below.

Disaster Syndrome

The average person directly involved in a disaster impact tends to
respond in a pattern which has been called the "disaster syndrome." This
disaster syndrome applies to the victims of the disaster, their immediate
families—whether injured or not—and some other persons who may have
been in the impact zone but who escaped injury. It does not refer to those
who come into the impact zone later.

Four stages have been recognized in the disaster syndrome. In the first
stage, which may last from minutes to hours after the impact, the person
is dazed, stunned, and apathetic. He cannot respond to directions. If told
to walk to an aid station, he may take one or two steps and then stop. He
may putter about the ruins of his home in a disorganized way, looking
for some trivial item, while disregarding a serious injury to himself or
a member of his family. The duration of this first stage can probably be
shortened by prior education in the ways to survive a disaster.

After anywhere from minutes to hours, depending on the individual,
the first stage gives way to the second. During the second stage, the person shows extreme suggestibility, altruism, and gratitude for help. He
tries to do whatever is asked of him, but his efficiency is low. If injured,
he is likely to minimize his own injuries and ask that others be taken care
of first. He is grateful that he is still alive. However, there may also be

the onset of guilt feelings because others did not survive and because he could not or did not help them. The second stage may last up to several days.

The third stage of the disaster syndrome is characterized by a mildly euphoric identification with the damaged community, a feeling of brotherhood with fellow sufferers, and enthusiastic participation in plans and activities for rebuilding. This stage may last for a few weeks.

The fourth stage includes increasing complaints, criticisms of agencies connected with disaster relief, and marked awareness of annoyance and loss. This stage gradually fades away as life returns to its normal patterns.

Panic

Panic is relatively rare in disasters but when it occurs, it can cause needless deaths and suffering. Panic can be defined as highly emotional behavior which is excited by the belief in an *immediate,* severe threat, and which results in actions that increase rather than decrease the danger for the individual and others. A key word here is "immediate." Panic does not ordinarily follow a warning of an impending threat which may not occur for an hour or more. However, some officials have refrained from giving early warning of a probable or possible disaster because of a misconception about the nature of panic, and because they were afraid such a warning might produce panic.

In the disasters which have been studied, panic occurred only when the following conditions existed:

1. There was a belief in an immediate severe danger—due in seconds or minutes.

2. There were a limited number of escape routes.

3. There was a belief that the escape routes were closing but were not yet closed.

4. There was no effective leadership and a lack of sound, correct information.

The actions of the average person in a disaster tend to be purposeful and sensible. He may flee—but flight in most cases is not panic. Since it usually lessens the danger, it is rational. Flight becomes panic only when it jams the exits and thus increases the dangers. Panic has on occasion resulted in panic-crushes, a situation that is described in greater detail in chapter 42.

The Volunteer Helper

The volunteer who goes into the impact area to help the victims also is changed by the disaster, and these changes should be understood if his services are to be used effectively and if he is to avoid becoming a hindrance or even an additional hazard. The volunteer helper, and by this we mean the untrained or semi-trained individual who rushes to the impact area, is subject to what has been called the "counter-disaster syndrome."

The Counter-Disaster Syndrome

The counter-disaster syndrome is found in some uninjured or slightly injured survivors of the impact and in many volunteers who come into the impact area to help. It is a relatively short-duration syndrome which is not usually divided into phases.

The counter-disaster syndrome is marked by extremely vigorous rescue activity. There is likely to be physical overexertion and the activity is relatively low in efficiency. Although the work performed has value, it is often done hastily and in a slipshod manner. Therefore, it must be checked by less emotionally involved persons. This, of course, applies particularly to first-aid measures. It should be pointed out that anyone can develop the counter-disaster syndrome, including nurses and doctors. The best preventive is education and training.

The volunteer helper also contributes in large part to the convergence problem. However, since this is caused by the sheer numbers of persons, rather than by their psychologic patterns, it is considered in chapter 9.

The Professional

The term "professional" used in this section refers primarily to full-time firemen and policemen, and to doctors, nurses, and other health maintenance persons who have had prior military training and experience. Doctors and nurses without any military background may, of course, adjust rapidly to the needs of the situation and behave in a fully professional manner, but not all are able to do so.

Studies of the responses of professionals to disasters show that, in general, they responded in an effective appropriate manner. They were able to evaluate the total situation correctly and apply their efforts where they did the most good. They were able in most cases to suppress personal anxieties and concentrate on getting the job done; this was accomplished often so quietly and efficiently that little attention was paid to them. Students of disasters have, in retrospect, decided that the roles of the professional firemen and policemen, for example, were greatly underestimated in the initial disaster studies.

The Onlooker

The onlooker at the disaster scene merely gets in the way of those who help the injured, making their tasks harder. In most American disasters, the number of onlookers and curious bystanders is so great as to constitute a major problem: convergence. This problem and ways of managing it are considered in chapters 9, 10, and 11. At this point, however, it is pertinent to consider the psychologic framework of these onlookers, aside from their effects on disaster management operations.

It has been customary for disaster workers, severely hampered by the curious, to refer to onlookers in such derogatory terms as "ghouls" and "thrill-seekers." Suggestions have been made that they be dealt with in a severe fashion, and rigid military discipline be imposed on the impact area. However, it has not proved feasible in the past to get enough National Guardsmen into the impact area rapidly enough to deal with all the onlookers in a military fashion. Other measures are needed, therefore, beginning with an understanding of the onlooker's psychology.

During the first hours after impact the distinction between volunteer worker and curious onlooker is far from clear. Many people who arrive as onlookers pitch in and perform valuable service as volunteers. On the other hand, many who come to the impact area as volunteer helpers find little to do in the area where they happen to be and become onlookers for lack of assignments.

Nevertheless, there are many people who come as onlookers and remain in that role. Most of these people are not ghouls or morbid thrill seekers. Instead, they are average people, with hidden anxiety about disasters. Some of them, perhaps, have guilt feelings because they have been spared while others were injured. In any event, their inner tension about the disaster forces them to view the impact area. They will go around roadblocks and detours and find ways of getting into the impact area. If properly directed, they are quiet and well-behaved. The act of viewing the disaster scene apparently helps them come to terms with their anxieties.

To be sure, in disaster management the major focus of our interest is the injured victim. The onlooker who gets in the way, even innocently, is a nuisance, and it is not advisable to expend any more effort or time on him than is absolutely necessary. However, it appears that the onlooker can be dealt with more rapidly and effectively by understanding and directing him than by attempting to institute repressive measures. These points are considered in greater detail in chapter 10.

chapter

5 EPIDEMIOLOGIC AND PUBLIC HEALTH ASPECTS OF DISASTERS

by Henry M. Parrish, M.D., Dr. P.H.

Epidemiology is concerned with the conditions under which diseases flourish. It may be referred to as the study of the "natural history" of disease. The word *epidemiology* is derived from the Greek terms *epi* (on or upon) and *demos* (the people), and implies a disease or a condition inflicted upon the people. Certainly a disaster is a condition suddenly thrust upon the people. The unit of study for the epidemiologist is a community (population group), whereas the unit of study for the medical practitioner is the individual person. Epidemiology is a basic science of public health and preventive medicine which aims towards the prevention of diseases and other injury-producing conditions.

The greatest disasters recorded in the history of mankind have been pandemics (unusually large and far-reaching epidemics) of infectious diseases such as the "Black Death" (plague), typhus fever, cholera, typhoid, smallpox, yellow fever and influenza *(see* chapter 31). Today these disastrous infectious diseases are largely prevented and controlled, due to an understanding of the epidemiology of the diseases, improvements in environmental sanitation, and other advances in medicine.

Most of the classical methods used in epidemiology resulted from studying infectious diseases. Following World War II, however, the epidemiologic method was used to study non-infectious diseases such as coronary heart disease, cancer, diabetes, arthritis, and mental diseases. Epidemiologists also have studied automobile, farm, home, and industrial accidents. Today, many injuries and deaths are prevented because we have identified and altered the causative factors associated with accidents. It seems probable that when the epidemiology of various kinds of disasters is known, many of them can be predicted and prevented, or at least controlled.

What are some of the epidemiologic factors associated with disasters? In most disasters there will be multiple causative factors. Epidemiologists have for convenience classified three types of factors which influence the incidence of a disease. They are:

20

1. *Agent factors.* The agent is the thing that produces the actual injury or disease.
2. *Host factors.* The hosts in disasters are human beings.
3. *Environmental factors.* The physical, chemical, biological and social climates in which a disaster happens.

Utilization of Epidemiologic Data and Approaches

The professional epidemiologist takes certain initial steps in investigating and dealing with an epidemic. In order to illustrate the manner in which these steps may be applied to any disaster, the following comparison is presented.

Epidemiologic Approach

Ordinary epidemic	Other disaster—an earthquake
1. Confirm the diagnosis.	Make sure the earthquake has occurred.
2. Determine if there is an epidemic.	Determine whether large numbers of people are injured or killed.
3. Characterize the epidemic according to time, place and person.	Find out when the earthquake occurred, the area involved, the number of people dead, missing, and injured, the amount of damage done, and the immediate needs of the survivors.

After the initial steps have been taken, some basic conclusions are drawn about the public health needs of the situation. The epidemiologic approach may next be used to determine in an orderly way the best ways to manage the problem. Each of the factors involved is systematically evaluated in order to discover the most effective method or methods of dealing with the disaster.

In order to illustrate the epidemiologic approach to a disaster, let us consider a disaster of substantial proportions which took place recently, and which has been studied fairly thoroughly.

An earthquake devastated part of the central plateau of Iran at 10:15 P.M. on September 1, 1962. There were about 150 villages and 150,000 persons in the disaster area. Approximately 12,000 persons were killed, 1,200 were seriously injured, and 30,000 families were left homeless.

I. Agent Factors

The primary causative agent was the earthquake itself. The agents causing deaths and injuries were collapsing buildings. The buildings were constructed of dried mud, tree trunks and twigs; they were not very resistant to earthquake damage. Fire was a minor agent, due to the lack of electricity and central heating in the houses. Secondary agents which provided a threat in the days and weeks following the earthquake were communicable diseases, malnutrition, and exposure to cold, since people lacked shelter. Delayed agents of disease came into play in the form of complications and chronic diseases among the injured.

Possible Preventive Measures

Primary agents. Nothing can be done to prevent earthquakes. Whether safer methods of house construction would be economically feasible, or even acceptable in this area of Iran, is not known. However, trained rescue workers and demolition experts could prevent additional injuries from collapse of damaged buildings.

Secondary agents. Communicable diseases can be controlled by environmental sanitation, pest control, establishment of an early reporting system, immunizations, and early isolation and treatment of the diseased.

Nutritional diseases can be prevented by providing essential foods, vitamins and minerals.

The harmful effects of exposure to cold may be prevented by supplying temporary shelters, clothing, blankets, fuel, and stoves.

II. Host Factors

Almost the entire population of the area was at risk of being killed or injured. Thus, both sexes and all age groups were involved. Approximately 12,000 people were killed and 1,200 were seriously injured. A few people who were sleeping outside were spared. Small infants were likely to become dehydrated and die if they were not rescued early. The same was true for people who were ill or injured or unable to help themselves. Fractures and crushing injuries to the head, chest and abdomen were the major types of injuries requiring medical care. In the period immediately after the disaster, psychological factors such as fright, confusion, anxiety and bereavement impaired self-help and rescue operations. Outside assistance to many villages was unavailable for several days. Some people were killed when they wandered into unsafe buildings, searching for their loved ones or possessions. Later, these people suffered additional physical stress from the lack of food, clothing and shelter. The educational level of the people was low and they had scanty knowledge about first aid. However, most of them were engaged in agriculture and they knew how to live off the land.

Possible Preventive and Corrective Measures

In the case of an earthquake, prior evacuation of the population is not possible because there isn't any real warning. The only practical solution for handling 12,000 dead at one time is mass burial, using bulldozers to dig large graves. Individual burial ceremonies must be abandoned. However, where possible, accurate lists of the dead should be kept.

Injured people should be handled by rescue, first aid, sorting, evacuation, initial medical treatment, definitive medical treatment and rehabilitation.

Living, uninjured people must be provided with food, clothing and shelter. Psychologic support may be given through good communications, efficient rescue, and opportunities to work in order to help their neighbors and themselves.

Special groups among the survivors may need special care. Infants will require milk; pregnant women will need provisions for childbirth, and chronically ill persons will need special medications.

III. Environmental Factors

A. *Physical environment.* The earthquake covered a geographic area of 23,000 square miles. Fortunately, it happened in a sparsely populated area; otherwise, the toll of human lives would have been much higher. Between 1904 and 1961, Iran had more than 115 major earthquakes. The terrain consisted of oases scattered among deserts and mountains. The closest medical center to the impact area was 90 miles away and Tehran, the capital of Iran, was 120 miles away. The lack of communications and paved roads to these isolated villages made rescue difficult. The temperature in the disaster area in September was that of dry heat during the days and extreme cold during the nights. Moreover, the freezing winter weather was only a few weeks away. The time of day that the earthquake struck (10:15 P.M.) increased the number of casualties. If the disaster had happened during the daylight working hours, fewer people would have been killed and these would have been predominantly women and children. Most of the homes were completely destroyed or rendered unsafe for habitation. Thus, shelter and clothing became a problem. Water, milk and food supplies were disrupted. No cold storage boxes were available to preserve perishable foods. Excreta disposal became a problem. Most of the livestock had perished in the quake since they were kept inside the mud houses at night.

B. *Chemical environment.* Insecticides were used for pest control and slaked lime was used as a disinfectant for excreta disposal and on decomposing bodies. These chemicals caused no problems.

C. *Biological environment.* The biological environment changed almost as drastically as the physical environment as a result of the disaster. The 12,000 people killed within a short period of time created an almost insurmountable burial problem. Furthermore, many dead human and animal bodies could not be excavated from the ruins for several days. This increased the possibility of a disease outbreak. Another problem was the identification of the dead and injured. There was about one seriously injured person for every 10 dead people. If the ratio of injured people had been higher there would have been increased demands on medical care personnel, supplies and facilities. The availability of food in the ruins provided an opportunity for disease-carrying rodents and insects to proliferate. The survivors of the earthquake were crowded into camps of tents and improvised shelters. A lack of clean water for drinking and bathing provided other hazards. People with various disease and immunization patterns were mixed together, especially when they were evacuated to larger cities. This mixing of susceptible people with diseased people is one of the best ways known to start and perpetuate epidemics of communicable diseases. Smallpox, typhus, typhoid, and tuberculosis are endemic in Iran. All of these diseases are capable of causing widespread epidemics.

D. *Social environment.* The earthquake disrupted community life, family life and personal life. The institutional framework of society was shattered. Established ways of doing things suddenly changed. Role positions were shifted. For example, community leaders and heads of families were lost; others had to take their places. These people worked in agriculture, had low per capita incomes and lived in small and medium-sized villages. Family activity, the home, farm land and livestock were important cultural values. The fact that livestock were housed with the family added to the loss.

The religious rite of ablution (washing the dead) had to be discontinued because of the overwhelming numbers of dead and the shortage of water. The general cultural view that the disaster was an act of fate probably retarded self-help and reconstruction. Although some seriously injured patients refused hospitalization, medical institutions were overrun by the sudden influx of large numbers of patients. Family life was upset by the loss of loved ones from death and injury. Many children became orphans. Some peasants had to migrate to large cities where they did not have the necessary skills to earn a livelihood. On the other hand, the country mobilized all of its resources to bring relief to the disaster victims. Other countries sent supplies and personnel to help these unfortunate people. No doubt the social and economic effects of this widespread disaster will be felt in Iran for many years to come.

Possible Preventive and Corrective Factors

Facilities for boiling water and provision of chlorine and iodine for chemical purification are needed. Water rationing may be necessary. Education of the survivors to the need of avoiding unsafe water may be essential. Because of the death of domestic animals, dried milk would be needed for infants. Adequate sewage, garbage and rubbish disposal are essential to keep down insects and rodents. Insecticides and rodenticides may also be required.

Every effort should be made to avoid mixing susceptible populations. Sick people should be isolated and treated promptly. People from different villages should not be mixed during evacuation or in temporary shelters.

Although the pre-existing social environment cannot be fully restored, the rehabilitation of the survivors is an important practical objective. Arrangements will be needed for future care of orphans, and for reuniting families separated by the disaster.

Conclusion

It will be noted that there is a certain degree of overlap and duplication in this approach. However, this helps prevent the omission of vital steps.

The epidemiologic approach to disaster is new, and alterations and modifications will undoubtedly be developed. It is hoped that through this or a similar approach, the accumulated knowledge and experience in epidemiology may be adapted and applied to the task of lessening the toll of all disasters.

chapter

6 ROLES AND ACTIVITIES IN DISASTER

This chapter describes the roles and activities carried out by different groups in helping disaster victims. It shows that there is a certain degree of overlap, and that some individuals will undertake additional activities even after their primary ones are completed.

In some cases, the activities performed by certain groups during past disasters corresponds closely to a theoretical optimal performance. In other cases, there have been serious discrepancies between what could have been done and what was actually done. The functions described, therefore, are those which are believed to contribute the most to the saving of lives and the relief of suffering.

Police

The police (and firemen) are usually the first to hear of a disaster and arrive upon the scene. They supply the information necessary for the organization of an orderly rescue and relief operation. First, the police should estimate the extent and character of the disaster and report it to the appropriate authorities. Subsequently, they will have a multitude of different tasks which must be performed efficiently if the total rescue operation is to function properly. Police radios can, in most cases, be used to set up a temporary communications system. The importance of this step is discussed in chapter 11. Also, a plan should be devised and put into operation at once for the direction and control of traffic into the impact area. The phenomenon of convergence, discussed in chapter 9, begins shortly after the impact. Unless a plan is devised to handle the traffic, the converging cars will jam the roads, making it exceedingly difficult to evacuate the injured or to get needed personnel and equipment into the area.

The police also take charge of the disaster scene unless and until relieved by superior authority. The extent to which the police exert a leadership role outside of strictly routine police duties will vary with the disaster training of the officers on the scene, with the nature of the disaster, and with the availability of other persons capable of leadership.

In most disasters it will not be advisable or practical for the police to attempt rescue or first-aid measures. Much more good will be done by handling the functions discussed here.

26

Firemen

The primary role of firemen in most disasters is the extinguishing and prevention of fires. In past disasters secondary fires have caused much greater damage and more deaths and injury than the initial disaster (*see* pp. 123, 135, and 156). In several cases, prompt action by firemen prevented small fires from developing into conflagrations or firestorms.* This role of the firemen is so vital that it should not be compromised by any other assignments or tasks, unless the firemen themselves are certain that all risk of fire is absent. In other words, it should have top priority over all other activities and in performing it, the firemen should be given complete cooperation by everyone at the disaster scene.

In disasters in which chemical agents are involved, firemen may undertake rescue roles because they are trained in the use of self-contained breathing apparatus and have such apparatus available.

Public Works Personnel

Personnel of public works departments should first perform any action which would lessen the chance of a secondary disaster. If the disaster has been one which breaks gas mains and power lines, all gas valves and electric power to the affected area should be turned off at once.

If roads have been blocked by debris, they should be cleared so that fire trucks can get through, followed later by other vehicles. If at any time the firemen require the use of heavy earth-moving equipment—such as bulldozers—to help fight a fire, such request should receive first priority.

Similarly, every possible assistance should be given to the firemen in obtaining adequate water supplies or anything else needed.

After the public works personnel have completed these tasks, they may undertake supervision of rescue operations, particularly of removing victims from under debris.

Civil Defense Personnel

Civil defense personnel should first coordinate their activities with those of the police and firemen. They should supply to the police and firemen any assistance which may be requested. Then, they should set up communications systems, first-aid stations, and rear-echelon collecting

---

* Robinson, D. *The Face of Disaster*. Doubleday, Garden City, N. Y., 1959, pp. 119-120.

Wallace, A. F. C. *Tornado in Worcester*. Disaster Study Number 3. National Academy of Sciences—National Research Council, Publication 392, Washington, D. C., 1956, p. 13.

points as described in chapters 9, 10, and 11. They should assist in organizing and directing the volunteer helpers in rescue, first aid and evacuation.

National Guard and Armed Forces

The primary role of the National Guard and armed forces should *not* be the prevention of looting. Actually, looting has been either nonexistent or minor in American disasters. It is a major waste of trained personnel to use the National Guard in this fashion. More effective roles for the Guard and armed forces are as follows:

1. Initially, assist police and firemen in their functions as needed.

2. Set up an *organized* pattern of communications, rescue, first aid, and evacuation, around which volunteers and trained professionals can base their own actions. A major deficiency in almost all disasters has been a lack of organization. Such organization could be developed rapidly on the site, in many cases, using Guard or armed forces units as cadres.

Doctors

The primary role of doctors should be to function as doctors. They should not be diverted into tasks, such as carrying stretchers, which can be done by ordinary volunteers. The role of an individual doctor will vary depending on his training and experience. Most surgeons should report to hospitals to perform surgery. However, to have several experienced surgeons at casualty collecting points to assign evacuation priorities to different types of casualties would be a great help.

Other physicians should set up first-aid stations and organize groups of volunteers as helpers.

Physicians who have had military or disaster training or experience could exert major leadership functions in organizing and directing large segments of the relief operation.

Nurses

Nurses may, depending on circumstances, take up a role as the doctor's main assistant and help, or they may function in a more independent fashion. Nurses can be of great help not only in the hospital but at the disaster site. In a large disaster there may be too few doctors for the number of first-aid stations needed. In such a situation, a nurse could set up and operate her own first-aid station. She should collect a group of volunteers and use them as assistants to the extent of their abilities.

A nurse with training or experience in disaster management could also assume additional leadership functions in organizing and directing major segments of rescue, first aid, and evacuation. It may be recalled that Florence Nightingale assumed similar leadership functions in an earlier disaster, the Crimean War. (*See* also Section II.)

Red Cross Personnel

The role of the Red Cross is to render assistance to local personnel in helping the victims of disaster. This assistance may be given in a multitude of ways, depending on the nature of the disaster and the degree of skill and training of local Red Cross personnel. In major disasters, experienced Red Cross personnel are usually flown to the site, but even so, early assistance must be given by local people. Some Red Cross groups can provide ambulance service; some can send well-trained first-aid teams to the impact area; most can provide such help as food, drink and temporary shelter for victims and rescuers. In addition, the national Red Cross office assumes a major responsibility for the rehabilitation of the disaster victims. The degree of interest in and support of the local Red Cross by the community bears a direct relationship to the extent of help which the local Red Cross can provide in a disaster.

Volunteers

In most disasters, volunteer helpers have provided the bulk of the rescue, first-aid and evacuation efforts. Unfortunately, their zeal has not been equalled by their experience, training or judgment. The activities of the volunteers, therefore, should be better controlled and be coordinated with those of professionally trained persons. This can best be accomplished if the volunteers would organize themselves into groups (like squads and sections), and place their services at the disposal of professionally trained persons. For example, a group of volunteers might help public works personnel rescue victims buried under debris. Other volunteers could help doctors and nurses run first-aid stations. Another group might organize a system for evacuation of casualties from first-aid stations to hospitals under the direction of doctors and civil defense personnel; still others could assist the police and firemen. In each case, the type of help given should correspond as closely as possible to the training and experience—including military—of the volunteer.

7 LEADERSHIP IN DISASTER

In any attempt to bring order and efficiency out of disorder and confusion, sound leadership is necessary. This is particularly true of disasters which are the epitome of disorder and confusion. Past experience has shown how helpful sound leadership can be, and how it can save lives and prevent suffering. By contrast, poor or absent leadership has sometimes resulted in needless extra casualties. In the discussion below we are concerned with leadership at all levels, not merely at one single supreme level.

The first principle to consider is that of practical goals. Any attempt to achieve the levels of leadership efficiency found in the military forces is bound to fail. However, a substantial degree of leadership efficiency can be attained, and can thus help to save lives and relieve suffering.

The second principle is that leadership in a disaster must be shared. Subordinate leaders in a disaster situation must be given a great deal of independent authority, or they are likely to be completely ineffective.

Another important principle is the organization of a leadership framework, or chain of command. The military model is excellent, provided one does not expect to achieve military efficiency levels.

The higher levels of leadership in a disaster should, ideally, be held by persons who already have recognized authority under existing law; for example: a Coast Guard officer, police chief, fire chief (unless he is needed to direct fire-fighting, which is more important), sheriff, mayor, civil defense director, National Guard commander, or a city manager.

Other persons qualified for high leadership roles are physicians and nurses with military experience, and active or retired military officers.

There should be no conflicts over leadership; "glory-hunting" must be avoided. In the event of conflict, it should be resolved at once.

It is appropriate to consider some of the qualities which fit a person to exercise sound leadership at a disaster.

There should be reasonably thorough knowledge about disasters. Knowledge of related fields is often helpful, but not always enough. The prospective leader should have the ability to teach quickly and effectively. He should be able to plan several steps in advance, and should be able to communicate with untrained people clearly, effectively and speedily.

He should understand the principles of organization, and of delegation of authority. Finally, experience in leadership would be of considerable help. Leadership should be an open-ended arrangement with both ends open. The first qualified person arriving on the scene takes charge of rescue, first aid and evacuation, organizing teams and groups, and appointing subordinate leaders. After some time has passed, he may notice that one of the subordinate leaders is highly competent and has good judgment. He may then ask the subordinate to take over, while he himself moves to another sector to repeat the process.

On the other hand, it may happen that a qualified person, after he has organized volunteer groups, encounters a later arrival on the scene who is better qualified as a leader than he is. He should then offer to turn the leadership of his group over to the better qualified person, while he assumes the position of assistant leader.

Another important leadership principle, which is especially applicable in a disaster, is identification of the leader. As Bowers and Hughes put it: "It would be much better if trained individuals could be identified in some way, since their assumption of control could be accepted. Trained individuals might well display the civil defense badges designating their special qualifications, but at the moment, such trained people are scarce."*

Some groups, fortunately, do have leadership symbols which are readily recognized by the average person. The best example is the nurses' white cap. It is, in addition, easily seen at a distance, even in poor light. A nurse, therefore, going to help at a disaster scene and wearing street clothes, should make every effort to bring and wear her cap. If it isn't possible to get one in time, it would be worthwhile to take a few minutes to fashion a makeshift cap from a handkerchief.

The higher-level leader at a disaster site would be well advised to appoint a nurse—in uniform, if possible, but at least with a cap—as a member of his immediate staff to remain close by his side. In that way, his leadership position would be clearly apparent to all, and his directives followed. The nurse herself could actually contribute much more by helping to bring order and organization to the confusion and chaos of the scene than by personally giving first aid.

At the lower levels of leadership, involving 12 persons or less, anyone may serve as a leader. There have been examples of excellent leadership by persons whose past training and experience did not seem particularly appropriate. After the Texas City explosion, a waitress assumed leadership

* Bowers, W. F. and Hughes, C. W. *Surgical Philosophy in Mass Casualty Management.* Charles C. Thomas, Springfield, Ill., 1960, p. 32.

of a group of volunteers, and did a creditable job of assisting the injured. Because of her white uniform everyone assumed she was a nurse. After the Flint tornado, a middle-aged kitchen helper came to the hospital to try to help. Since no one assigned her a task, she looked around for one. She heard that soiled operating-room linen was piling up, so she called in friends and neighbors and organized them, and they washed the soiled linen, preparing it for sterilization.

During a disaster, anyone who remotely reminds the population of a leadership figure will usually be able to collect a nucleus of volunteer assistants. Women in white uniforms, of course, resemble nurses and are likely to be obeyed by volunteers. In addition, men with peaked caps— like milkmen and delivery men—have been asked to lead because their caps, worn also by policemen and soldiers, conveyed an aura of leadership.

The question of local vs. outside leadership has arisen in many disasters. Usually, that part of the local population which is uninjured feels a great need to do something to help their neighbors. Those who have had leadership roles in the community tend to feel threatened by the presence of outside experts. They may, subconsciously, fear that they will lose their opportunity to make good before the world. These are normal human feelings which are quite understandable. Nevertheless, the history of civil disasters has shown that "usually an outside individual or agency has to come into the area and assume control before things begin to move. Partly this is because local disruption of organization paralyzes action, and partly it is because there is no one locally who is recognized as the chosen leader. . . ."* The problem is that a conflict between local and outside groups over leadership might seriously interfere with effective aid.

A capable leader should be able to resolve this situation diplomatically and without any undue waste of time. The use of appropriate titles can be most helpful in some cases. For example, a trained, capable leader coming in from the outside after a moderate disaster need not call himself the leader. Instead, he can arrange with some local official to serve as his "advisor," "consultant," "chief of staff," etc.

At the higher leadership levels, the staff system, which has worked so well in military situations, should be used. The person in charge of a disaster area should collect and assign as his staff the best qualified people who are immediately available. If better qualified persons come along later, substitutions or additions may be made. The staff arrangement should be flexible. It may be helpful to present the authors' concept of an effective

* *Ibid.,* p. 32.

staff system at a moderate disaster, involving about 100 deaths and about 1,000 seriously injured. It is as follows:

1. *Chief of staff.* He is responsible for finding and helping to appoint, assign and direct members of the staff. This should be someone with some military training.

2. *Area safety officer.* He is responsible for prevention of any further casualties in the disaster area. For example, he should make sure that there is no danger of fire or explosion, of a return of a tornado, a second tsunami, collapse of a weakened building, etc. He should keep informed of all factors which might endanger victims and rescuers. At any time that he believes a danger to exist, he should warn the commander directly. He need not consult with the chief of staff. Furthermore, he should have absolute priority in the use of all communications facilities. The area safety officer should be the person with the best knowledge of disasters. If there had been an effective area safety officer at the Texas City explosion of 1949, the death toll would have been ten or less instead of 561. (*See* p. 136).

3. *Executive officer.* He should be responsible for transmitting all orders and directives from the overall commander to the subordinate commanders.

4. *Communications officer (rear).* He would be in charge of setting up and maintaining lines of communication between the disaster headquarters and hospitals, depots, and other areas outside the impact zone. He may use whichever methods are available to him.

5. *Communications officer (forward).* He would be in charge of setting up and maintaining communications with disaster teams and groups in the impact area. Probably he will have to rely upon runners or bicyclers for the most part.

6. *Traffic control officer.* Preferably, he should be an officer of the highway patrol.

7. *Heavy rescue officer.* He makes arrangements to get heavy rescue equipment—cranes, bulldozers, etc.—into the area. He should be an engineer or contractor, if possible.

8. *Supply officer.* He should coordinate all requests for supplies from the disaster teams and arrange to have those supplies obtained and delivered at the earliest possible moment.

9. *Medical liaison officer.* His duties should include keeping in touch with the hospitals, finding out their capacities to handle emergency cases, and routing casualties to those hospitals that have the greatest unused capacity. In some cases, the hospitals in the area may not have the ability

to handle all the injured in a reasonable period of time. In that event, many of the casualties would have a much better chance of recovery if evacuated to more distant areas (*see* chapter 14). The medical liaison officer should be prepared to advise the overall commander when and how this should be done. The medical liaison officer may be a physician, nurse, or medical administrator.

8 ORGANIZATION OF DISASTER TEAMS

A major lesson to be learned from our past experiences with disaster is the high cost of disorganization. Every effort should be made to organize the efforts to help the victims. Such organization would be invaluable if it could be done before the impact of the disaster. To a limited extent, groups and teams which could provide coordinated help to disaster victims are being formed. These groups are usually based on local civil defense organizations.

There is also a promising field in industry for organizing volunteer evacuation, rescue and first-aid teams, just as there are now industry-sponsored basketball, baseball, and bowling teams. If such groups could be set up, trained, and equipped, they could provide valuable service in disasters within 50 miles of their plant location. An industrial physician or nurse associated with a particular company could take the initiative in organizing, training and leading various types of disaster teams which would be ready to function as soon as a disaster occurred.

In the forseeable future, however, the bulk of the help in disasters will be rendered by volunteers who come as individuals and small groups to the impact area. The effectiveness of their help can be increased manyfold by proper direction and organization. A professionally trained person could, in a matter of minutes, organize these volunteers into teams and give them enough basic direction and supervision to improve the handling of the situation greatly.*

Let us consider some examples of teams which could be set up, their functions, and suggested structure.

I. Light Rescue Team

A. *Mission:* to rescue injured persons who are covered with light debris which does not require sawing, metal-cutting, or heavy equipment.

B. *Equipment:* hand-tools, as available.

C. *Personnel:*

1. Leader—any person with a clear head and some leadership experience, such as a schoolteacher, foreman, veteran, or minister.

2. Assistant leader.

* Lueth, H. C., Emergency Medical, Hospital, and Nursing Care. *Ann. Amer. Acad. Pol. and Soc. Sci., 309:* 142, Ja. 1957.

3. Rescuemen—six to ten volunteers in reasonably good health—to remove debris from victims.

4. Couriers (two) to bring first-aid teams to victims who have been rescued and to get help from heavy rescue teams where necessary.

II. Heavy Rescue Team

A. *Mission:* to rescue injured persons who are covered with heavy debris, requiring sawing, metal-cutting, or heavy lifting equipment (i.e., cranes, pulleys, etc.).

B. *Equipment:* wood- and metal-cutting tools; power equipment as available.

C. *Personnel:*

1. Leader—preferably an engineer, architect, or building contractor.

2. Assistant leader.

3. Six to 12 skilled workmen who know how to use the tools available.

4. Couriers (two) to arrange interchanges of scarce equipment. (For example, one team may have a crane which is not in immediate use, while another team a few blocks away needs a crane.)

III. First-Aid Team

A. *Mission:* to provide first aid to the injured where they lie, before evacuation, so as to prevent further injury during evacuation.

B. *Equipment:* whatever may be available—probably very little.

C. *Personnel:*

1. Leader—nurse, nursing student, medical student, dentist, pharmacist, and other health-team personnel.

2. Assistant leader.

3. Two splint quartermasters—whose duties include obtaining or making crude splints and bandages from debris in the area and furnishing them to the first-aid men.

4. First-aid men—six persons with some prior first-aid training. Examples are boy scouts, girl scouts, veterans, and citizens who have satisfactorily completed civil defense or Red Cross first-aid courses.

5. Three couriers—to direct litter bearers to splinted victims who are ready for transportation to collecting points.

IV. Litter Team

A. *Mission:* to transport the injured to a medical collecting point after first aid has been given.

B. *Equipment:* whatever may be available. Litter bearers will make own litters from debris.

C. *Personnel:*

1. Leader—any person with a clear head and some leadership experience. Examples are schoolteachers, foremen, veterans, ministers.
2. Assistant leader.
3. Litter bearers (15 men) organized into three squads of five men each, including the squad leader. These men should be in good health and relatively strong.
4. Three couriers to find best routes to medical collecting points and to direct litter bearer squads.

V. Communications Team

A. *Mission:* to set up communications in the impact area and between the impact area and supporting facilities, such as hospitals and medical collecting points.

B. *Equipment:* where possible, two-way radios in vehicles; a network of taxicabs would be excellent.

C. *Personnel:*
1. Leader—a policeman, civil-defense official, military or civilian officer.
2. Assistant leader.
3. Communications men—six to ten persons in vehicles equipped with two-way radios who know how to use the equipment.
4. Assistant communications men—six to ten volunteers, assigned one to each vehicle as assistants to help in any way necessary, including serving as couriers if required.

In some situations, other teams could be organized for special purposes. For example, if firemen needed help, auxiliary fire teams could be organized on the spot and put at the disposal of the firemen. The organization of the teams as outlined above is merely a series of suggested examples. Other structures may work as well or better in some disasters.

There are a number of basic principles to keep in mind in organizing such teams.

First, in the confusion of a disaster no person can direct more than ten helpers efficiently unless there are intermediate leaders. In general, no person who has not had extensive military command experience can direct more than three subordinate leaders.

In organizing teams and groups of teams, the principle of open-ended organizations at top and bottom should be followed. That is, each team should be ready to incorporate additional volunteers until the size exceeds ten persons per leader. Then the team is split into two teams, with the assistant leader taking over one, and two new assistant leaders being appointed.

If the team leader encounters another trained professional whom he considers better qualified, he should turn leadership of the team over to that person and become an assistant leader until the team becomes large enough to split into two. For example, a first-year medical student might organize and direct a first-aid team. If a fourth-year medical student then arrives in the area, it would be proper to offer to turn over team leadership to him.

It is important to give clear, simple assignments to the volunteer helpers; under the stress of a disaster, the chances of misunderstanding are much greater than in normal life. The leader should not ordinarily attempt to do much of the work himself. Instead, his time will be most effectively used in close supervision of his subordinates. At times, however, the team leader may have to demonstrate a certain procedure to the members of the team.

The organization of the disaster team should be started at the earliest moment. If it is possible to organize a team before a disaster occurs, that much the better. The next best thing is to organize the team *before* going into the impact area, and travel together into the area. If bus or truck transportation of volunteers into the impact area is available, the teams can be organized while riding to the scene, and some preliminary instructions can be given then. Traffic checkpoints and roadblocks also are good places to organize teams. Finally, teams can be organized right in the impact area in about two or three minutes, and some of the needed directions can be given while rescue work is actually going on.

After a disaster team is organized and has started work, the leader may send a courier to look for a person in authority who will accept the responsibility of directing several sets of teams.

9 CONVERGENCE IN DISASTERS

Convergence is the movement of persons and materials into the impact area from the periphery. The movements requested or ordered by agencies or authorities with official disaster responsibilities are generally a very small fraction of the total movement into the area. Most of the convergence is unofficial.

In past disasters unofficial convergence has been one of the greatest obstacles to giving efficient help to the victims. The extent to which convergence hampers effective rescue, first aid, and evacuation is usually much greater than most people realize. It is important, therefore, to understand the convergence phenomenon, its origins, and possible ways of dealing with it.

First, let us consider a few examples of convergence of persons in past disasters and get some idea of the magnitude of the problem.

1. A tornado struck White County, Arkansas, on March 21, 1952. Within an hour, hundreds of automobiles began moving into the impact area. This flow of traffic continued for *over a week*. By 10 A.M., on Sunday, cars were lined up bumper to bumper for ten miles on each side of the disaster center. It required, in addition to local police, 80% of the highway patrol of the *entire state* to unsnarl the traffic jam. In many cases, emergency vehicles could not get into or out of the impact area. Note that this took place in an area which was not heavily populated by eastern standards.

2. After the Waco, Texas, tornado of May 11, 1953, the entire downtown area became jammed with traffic. The following Sunday, many more people came. Airplanes buzzed over the ruins, creating sky traffic jams. The police chief of Waco estimated that at one large intersection alone, 10,000 people were standing, doing nothing constructive, and stopping progress so that trucks had to proceed through the crowd at a snail's pace.

3. In December 21, 1951, there was a mine explosion in West Frankfort, Illinois. Cars began coming in to the community, reaching a peak of 1,000 cars per hour.

4. In 1951, there was an explosion and a fire in a chemical plant in Charleston, West Virginia. Within ten minutes, every road leading to the plant was completely jammed with cars. As a result, fire-squad members

and other professional personnel had to leave their vehicles three to four miles away and carry their equipment that distance to help put out the fire. Most American motorists are familiar with traffic jams. However, those in and around disaster areas are usually far worse than ordinary holiday tie-ups. The reason is that after a disaster, roads leading to the impact area from all directions become so clogged that it soon becomes virtually impossible to detour or reroute traffic.

The convergers usually start descending on a disaster area as soon as the first reports are given on radio and television. The convergence continues for a variable period, depending on the size and nature of the disaster, the location, time of year, and other factors. In some cases, convergence has continued for over a week.

The convergence phenomenon has several origins. Fritz and Mathewson* have classified the convergers into five major types:

The returnees. These are people who live in the disaster area and either were away at the time of impact or had received minor injuries which were cared for. These people are a small fraction of the total.

The anxious. These are usually relatives of the impact area's inhabitants. They are worried about their loved ones and seek to learn their fate. These people are a moderate fraction of the total at the impact area but a major part of the total at hospitals. They present problems in handling, since they cannot be stopped by ordinary police measures such as roadblocks. The extent of their anxiety is usually such that they seek to find ways around all obstacles.

The helpers. These people actually have performed a major part of the rescue and evacuation work in past disasters.

The curious. The motivation of these people has been discussed in chapter 4.

The exploiters. These people form a numerically insignificant minority of the convergers, although their activities can be quite a nuisance.

The basic problem in handling the convergence crowds is not that they are disorderly, unlawful, or unruly, but that the sheer volume of persons and automobiles is too great to handle with the trained personnel available or in the limited road space of the disaster area. In the past several errors have been made in trying to handle disaster convergence.

* Fritz, C. E. and Mathewson, J. H. *Convergence Behavior in Disaster: A Problem in Social Control.* Disaster Study Number 9. National Academy of Sciences—National Research Council, Publication 476, Washington, D. C., 1957.

First, local governmental officials have seriously underestimated the extent of convergence which was building up, and greatly overestimated their own ability to handle converging crowds.

Second, usual routine traffic control procedures were applied to the converging crowds without enough thought about their applicability. For example, if at the onset of a disaster the main roads are blocked off, convergers do not simply go home—they find the side roads and clog those. Traffic jams develop on the main roads before the road blocks are reached. By that time, any attempt to route emergency vehicles over secondary roads is likely to fail because they, too, are already jammed.

Also, too much faith was put in the effectiveness of radio and television appeals to stay away from the area. These did not work, and seem to have little promise of ever working.

In some cases convergence was made much worse by thoughtless appeals for help on radio or television. After the Flint-Beecher (Michigan) tornado of June 8, 1953, rescue work was hampered by a shortage of flashlights. A request for flashlights was broadcast, and 500 people who might otherwise have stayed home responded by driving 500 cars—containing one flashlight each—into the already jammed disaster area. One or two vehicles could easily have carried the needed flashlights.

In the same disaster someone broadcast an appeal for blood donors which the hospitals didn't need or want. Two thousand extra people then jammed the hospitals, trying to donate their blood.

Thus far, we have considered the problem of personnel convergence in terms of hindering the rescue work. There is, however, an additional hazard to convergence which, in some disasters, is much more serious: the convergers themselves may become victims of a secondary disaster. As pointed out in chapter 1, this was the case in the Texas City explosion.

Shortly after the impact area begins to fill up with crowds, a second wave of convergers starts to jam the hospitals in the area. These hospital convergers come for a variety of reasons, most of them legitimate and praiseworthy. Some who have special skills come to volunteer their services. Others come because of anxiety about loved ones who are missing; they wander about, looking for the missing persons. Still others come to offer blood. Despite the good intentions, however, the net effect of the sheer volume of persons coming into a small area is a marked hindrance to the work of helping the injured.

At about the same time, another type of convergence sets in, jamming the communications channels. Telephone calls swamp hospital switchboards, so that essential calls—both incoming and outgoing—cannot be made. Any other agency associated with the disaster is also swamped with calls.

A few days later, still another type of convergence, although of much less importance, adds to the difficulties in rehabilitating the disaster area. Kind-hearted persons throughout the nation donate old clothing and other material to the stricken area. Some of the donated material has real value, much of it does not. The job of sorting, distributing, and storing the donations is often a severe strain on community resources.

There have so far been few examples of sound, effective ways of handling the convergence problem. In no case which we have come across have local authorities been able to act quickly and effectively enough to prevent, or significantly reduce, the immediate convergence on the impact area. Similarly, we are unaware of any hospital which has managed to keep the convergers from disrupting its disaster plan in a major disaster. There have, however, been a few cases in which a workable plan was devised by police officials to manage late convergence of personnel (several days after the initial impact). The cars of convergent sightseers were channeled along a planned route to enable them to view the damage, and then get out of the area rapidly. In effect, this amounted to a kind of guided tour. Of course, some persons may object to such an arrangement and consider it unethical or even immoral to help the sightseers satisfy their curiosity. They may prefer a strict, punitive method of handling the convergers, with rather rigid prohibitions placed on them. However, this attitude is based on some misconceptions about the psychology of the sightseers (*see* chapter 4).

It appears that the best way to handle the problem is empirically, i.e., by determining which approach works best, not which is most satisfying to the emotional needs or the moral sense of the persons in authority. Those who have studied the problem have concluded that convergence cannot be blocked but it can be channeled. The channeling of late convergers into a guided tour does work and reduces markedly the hindrance to effective disaster management.

It may be possible in some cases to apply similar principles to the early convergers, and thus reduce the extent to which they interfere with rescue operations. Some suggestions for accomplishing this are presented in chapter 10; methods of handling convergence on hospitals are discussed in chapters 15 and 16.

10 TRAFFIC CONTROL

The importance of traffic control in and around a disaster scene should become clear when one considers the convergence problems of past disasters. This chapter, therefore, will discuss some ways of improving traffic control operations in a disaster area.

Before an effective traffic control system can be put into operation, a basic plan should have been worked out in advance and should be understood by those who will have to apply it.

The most logical group to draft and execute such a plan would be the highway patrol (or state police). The plan should be drawn up with the cooperation of state civil defense officials, and should provide for assistance to the highway patrol by civil defense auxiliary police and police from nearby towns. Existing state laws should be modified, if necessary, bestowing state-wide authority on city police and auxiliaries when working under the supervision and direction of a highway patrol officer.

Some elements of a sample plan will be presented after certain other basic points have been considered.

A major requirement for an effective traffic control plan is speed in setting it up, since often, within ten minutes of the disaster impact, roads to this area are so filled with cars that police vehicles have difficulty getting to their posts. One way to avoid this has been suggested which holds considerable promise. This would be an agreement, worked out voluntarily and well in advance, with all radio and television stations in the state, to put a 30-minute delay on initial flash bulletins about a disaster which has already occurred. (This would, of course, not apply to warnings about an impending disaster.) This 30-minute grace period would give the highway patrol time to set up its traffic control plan, as well as get essential rescue teams moved into the area. An argument can be advanced that a 30-minute delay in the announcement would also mean a delay in moving rescuers into the area. This would be true of a small number of people, such as doctors who are driving along in their cars with their radios playing. The movement of the bulk of the important rescue personnel, however, would not be slowed down, since they would be alerted by hospitals, Red Cross, etc. These professionally trained persons are not likely to be sitting around, listening to the radio or watching television during the times when most disasters strike. The benefits to be gained by having enough time to set up a traffic control plan would far outweigh the minor loss of not alerting an occasional doctor who happens to be listening to the radio.

Furthermore, the 30-minute delay would not result in a serious shortage of untrained volunteer helpers. The people in the filter area (see chapter 3) would know of the disaster as soon as it strikes, and would move to the impact area without any announcements. Their convergence would be a minor problem, and they could form the pool of unskilled manpower during the first 30 minutes.

The argument might also be raised that a radio or television flash would alert parents about the need of rescuing their children, or a husband about his wife's peril, and that a delay would be unfair to them. However, this argument also is invalid. A coordinated rescue operation would help the victims much more rapidly and effectively than the frantic efforts of relatives. The notification of relatives via radio and television would also result in the notification of hordes of curious sightseers who would cause a tremendous traffic jam (chapter 9). Indeed, there is every likelihood that if there is enough delay in the radio and television announcements to allow the setting up of a traffic control system, the anxious relatives would arrive at the disaster scene *sooner* than if the announcement were made at once.

If the announcement were made immediately, the victims' relatives might start out 30 minutes earlier, but due to the traffic jam might be delayed many hours in reaching the impact area. With the proposed delay, however, they would start 30 minutes later and arrive much sooner.

Another important consideration is the fact that there will probably be little, if any, parking space in the impact area, and that what there is, will be needed for police and fire vehicles, ambulances, and heavy rescue equipment. A traffic control plan, therefore, should include a stipulation that private vehicles, entering the impact area, cannot park there but must discharge their passengers and move on. Exceptions should be made only for physicians, nurses, and high-ranking governmental and civil defense personnel. Parking areas well away from the impact area could be used, if available.

The next point to remember is that restrictive measures do not work well in disaster situations. It would be nice if they did, but experience shows otherwise. Convergence cannot be blocked; it must be channeled.

This means that the plan should also include provisions to keep traffic moving.

One device that has been applied in most disasters, but could be applied more effectively, is the sorting of traffic. This works as follows: at a road-block or diversion point, important rescue traffic—such as cranes, ambulances, doctors, nurses, and civil defense personnel—is passed through directly to the impact area, while most other traffic is routed, at a lower speed, along a succession of country side-roads so as to arrive much later. Residents of the impact area, trying to locate their families, can be directed to a diversion point and allowed to use the direct route with the emergency vehicles, thus more than making up the 30-minute delay.

Let us now consider a sample plan for traffic control in a disaster. It must be understood that this plan is only a sample, that it is incomplete, and that it would have to be modified and expanded to fit the needs of a particular state. It is based on the assumption that the radio and television stations have agreed to delay the news of the disaster by 30 minutes. Without that grace period, a far more complex plan would be needed.

I. Highway Patrol

A. The first highway patrol vehicle to reach the general vicinity of the disaster proceeds as far as possible into the heart of the impact area, radioing information to headquarters on the estimated damages and casualties and the names of streets involved. The vehicle halts and assumes a semi-permanent station either on reaching the heart of the impact area, or on being blocked by impassable debris. The patrolman may organize survivors and volunteers into disaster teams, but he himself remains with his vehicle. The vehicle should become a forward command and communications post.

B. If the patrolman (or headquarters) believes there is a danger of a secondary impact, then his vehicle becomes more important as a warning device than as a communications point. In that case, he cruises the area and uses a loudspeaker to warn of a possible secondary impact.

C. In large disasters, a secondary highway patrol vehicle, approaching from another direction, may be sent in.

D. Subsequent highway patrol vehicles are assigned stations at road junctions from five to 15 miles away from the impact area. A partial roadblock is set up just beyond the intersection.

For the first 30 minutes—until the radio and television announcement of the disaster—traffic is allowed to pass unhindered, unless it appears to be excessively heavy to the officer at the scene. Municipal police, sheriffs, deputies, or civil defense auxiliary police arriving at the intersection are to be halted and assigned as assistants to the highway patrolman. These assistants are to be directed in forming an efficient sorting system to go into effect when traffic increases (*see* E below); up to eight assistants may be needed at each intersection. If another police vehicle, with a *uniformed* officer and a radio powerful enough to reach the nearest headquarters, arrives at the intersection, the highway patrolman may be directed to turn the responsibility for the intersection over to him, and to report to another site.

E. Until more specific orders arrive from headquarters, the sorting of traffic will begin after the 30-minute grace period or when traffic seems excessively heavy. In the sorting process, the following vehicles will be sent through directly to the impact area:

1. Fire vehicles (top priority).
2. Electric and power company vehicles.
3. Telephone company vehicles.
4. Civil defense directors.
5. Military vehicles.
6. Construction vehicles (i.e., cranes, bulldozers, etc.).
7. Buses with volunteer helpers.
8. Trucks suitable for carrying litters.
9. Physicians (even if one to a car).
10. Nurses (even if one to a car).
11. Any vehicle with a two-way radio.
12. Off-duty highway patrolmen or other police or fire officers (even if one to a car).

The above groups will, in general, be permitted to park in or near the disaster area.

In addition, persons belonging to the categories below should be allowed to use the main route until contrary orders are sent from higher headquarters. These vehicles will not be allowed to park in or near the impact area; they must discharge passengers, and either pick up casualties at once or leave for a parking area well outside of the impact zone.

13. Volunteer disaster teams with not less than six persons per vehicle including the driver, or a lesser number of persons, if accompanied by important supplies.
14. Persons who claim to be residents of the disaster area. Their license number should be written down, and they should be told that their claim will be checked. This maneuver is designed to discourage sightseers from using a falsehood in order to gain access to the area.

15. Persons with specially relevant training (i.e., explosives experts, engineers, etc.) who can identify themselves.

F. Other vehicles will be routed along secondary roads.

G. Homemade signs, megaphones, or any other devices may be used to improve the efficiency of the sorting process.

H. All speed limits are to be strictly observed by all vehicles without exception, especially ambulances.

II. Highway Patrol Headquarters

The following steps should be instituted simultaneously:

A. All off-duty patrolmen are to be alerted for emergency duty and some asked to report.

B. Some patrol vehicles in other parts of the state are to move toward the disaster area.

C. The following are to be notified of the disaster at once:

1. Civil defense headquarters.

2. All hospitals in the area and those outside the area which might receive casualties.

3. The Red Cross.

4. National Guard headquarters—so that initial preparations can be made for rapid assembly, should they be called up.

5. Police and fire chiefs in towns and villages within a 25 to 50 mile radius of the impact area. Fire-fighting equipment may be the greatest need.

D. A tentative traffic-routing plan should be drawn up and radioed to the appropriate patrol cars within five minutes, including this information:

1. Main routes for emergency vehicles.

2. Roadblock points.

3. Detour routes for vehicles of low priority.

4. Collection points outside the impact area where volunteers can meet and consolidate their transportation, so as to reduce vehicular traffic into the impact zone.

chapter

11   COMMUNICATIONS

An adequate communication system would be a major factor in reducing the confusion and disorganization at the disaster scene, and at the supporting facilities. In almost all past disasters, communications were grossly inadequate, so that it proved virtually impossible to coordinate efforts to help the victims. In one disaster, there was a great need for a crane to help rescue victims from under debris. A crane of the proper sort stood idle a few blocks away, but because of lack in communications no one knew about it. Hospitals are usually subjected to a great deal of confusion because of inadequate communications with the impact area and with other hospitals.*

Let us first consider the strategic points between which communications should be established and maintained, and then the methods which may be used to accomplish this. The following areas should be able to communicate with each other:

1. The impact area and the forward command post. If the impact area is large, it may be necessary to divide it into sectors, with each sector reporting to the command post.

2. The forward command post with:

    a. Impact area.

    b. Medical collection point.

    c. Rear command post, if one has been set up.

    d. Highway patrol headquarters.

    e. State civil defense headquarters.

    f. At least one hospital or medical facility in the rear area.

3. The medical collecting point with:

    a. Forward command post.

    b. Hospitals.

4. Hospitals with:

    a. Command posts.

    b. Every other hospital in the area.

    c. Highway patrol headquarters.

---

* Raker, J. W. *et al. Emergency Medical Care in Disasters.* National Academy of Sciences—National Research Council, Washington, D. C., 1956, p. 44.

d. Local municipal police headquarters.

e. State and local civil defense headquarters.

The means of establishing communications will vary with each situation. In the impact area, telephone communication will probably be impossible for some time. The following methods can be used instead:

1. Two-way radios in police cars and other vehicles.
2. Couriers on bicycles or on foot.

If a command post is set up at the outskirts of the disaster area—near the fringe area—telephone communication to the rear may be available. If only a single telephone is available, it should be reserved for essential calls and under no circumstances be released to newspapermen, etc. The most efficient use of one or a few telephones would be to maintain *continuous* contact with an agency in the rear, which would relay information on *other* phones to other agencies. For example, if important messages are to be sent to the state highway patrol, civil defense, and four or five hospitals, it would be a waste of time to try and talk to each in turn. Their switchboards would most likely be swamped with calls, and it may take hours to get through. To make contact with one agency, instead, and preferably with the highway patrol, would keep the lines open at both ends for the duration of the emergency. Messages for civil defense and the hospitals would then be given to the highway patrol, who, through other phones, by radio, or if necessary by messenger, would relay them to the other agencies.

If an operable telephone is not available near the disaster area, messages can be relayed by vehicles equipped with two-way radio. These messages should be simple and direct and worded carefully to avoid mix-ups in the relay procedure.

In areas outside the impact zone, telephone communication should, in theory, be a practical means of communication. However, in past disasters, the flood of incoming calls to civil defense headquarters and hospitals has usually jammed all switchboards so that even outgoing calls were difficult or impossible to complete; communication from hospital to hospital by telephone was often impossible. There is not much that can be done to remedy this, once a disaster strikes. However, a little advance planning can solve this problem readily.

Each hospital should have at least one unlisted telephone line, independent of its switchboard, preferably in the office of the director or the chief nurse. The number of this line should be made known to other hospital directors, highway patrol and civil defense headquarters, who, in turn, agree not to divulge it to any unauthorized persons and to use it only for essential disaster communication. It should be borne in mind, though, that a single line, while much better than nothing, is hardly enough to maintain communications to and from a hospital during a disaster.

Another scheme is worth mentioning. Most hospitals have coin telephones for the convenience of patients and visitors. These telephones do not go through the switchboard, and therefore are not likely to be jammed with incoming calls. (However, in some past disasters, they have been usurped by newspapermen.) It would be well to make a listing of these telephone numbers, and exchange these lists between all hospitals in the area, and highway patrol and civil defense headquarters. When a disaster strikes, two hospital employees should be assigned to each coin telephone, with orders to pre-empt and reserve it for essential hospital communications; one employee stays with the telephone all the time while the other acts as a courier. If the communications load is light, the hospital director may allow the general public limited use of these phones.

If arrangements have been made beforehand, these telephones can be used to set up a rather efficient network. One phone can be assigned to the nursing service, one to the chief of surgery, etc. Alternatively, a communications service can be set up with the phones receiving messages for and sending messages from a central message center. There should be no question of the advisability of assigning hospital employees to these coin telephones. Those assigned can be people working in the business office, in personnel, and other areas which are not essential to emergency patient care. The value of maintaining an effective communications system would far outweigh the loss of services of a few employees in these categories.

The possibility must also be considered that the disaster may destroy all telephone communications in a large area, including the hospitals. To guard against this eventuality, a short-wave two-way radio network would be invaluable. The frequencies used should be coordinated so that the various hospitals can communicate with each other, and with the highway patrol and civil defense headquarters. Usually, the local civil defense director is of great help in these arrangements, and, in many cases, he is able to obtain superior radio equipment at a marked reduction in cost.

In most disasters, radio amateurs have been of great help in relaying important messages. It can be anticipated that they will continue to provide important communications assistance, in every way possible. It would be preferable, though, for hospitals to have their own radio equipment, and not have to rely on help from radio hams.

There is another aspect of the communications problem which should be considered—communication to the general public. This may be divided into two parts; communications about the total disaster, and communications about individual victims. In most past disasters, communications about the total disaster were left to the judgment of those who are in charge of radio and television stations. These people, although well-meaning, have had little or no training in disaster problems and as a result, their attempts to help have often resulted in greater confusion. The classic example of getting 500 automobiles, each carrying one flashlight, to move into an already jammed impact area has already been mentioned. Since ordinary news bulletins on the disaster tend to promote convergence, the best solution would be to educate radio and television personnel in disaster problems. If this proves not to be practical, another possible, partial solution would be to give careful consideration to all disaster information and messages disseminated by radio or television. For example, if flashlights are needed at the impact zone, the message should not be to "bring flashlights" but, instead, it should ask that flashlights be taken to schools and churches nearest the homes of the donors; there they could be collected and dispatched to the rescuers in one school or church car.

Communications about individual victims have, in the past, resulted in serious problems for hospitals. Hospital switchboards are not designed to handle the enormous volume of incoming calls that can be expected after a disaster. A partial solution would be to set up an information center in a building outside the hospital—such as a nurses' residence—preferably one with a large switchboard. In some cases, it may be possible for the telephone company to provide temporary emergency switchboard service. The information center can be staffed with volunteers who maintain listings of patients and their conditions, supplied by couriers at regular intervals. By using this sort of device, some of the jamming of hospitals' switchboards can be avoided. Advance planning, too, can help prevent confusion and inefficiency.

12 RESCUE

The term "rescue" as used in disaster involves two related types of activity. One type of rescue is the removal of persons from a dangerous location to one of safety. Examples are rescuing shipwreck survivors and persons in burning buildings. This type of rescue operation is usually handled by trained professionals and often requires special equipment. The details of the procedures involved do not come within the scope of this book.

The other type of rescue involves the finding and freeing of persons trapped by debris, whether they are injured or not. This phase of rescue operations is ordinarily handled by volunteers who may or may not have any pertinent training or knowledge. In many past disasters the untrained volunteer rescuers did things in such a manner as to increase the danger to the victims and to themselves.* Therefore, it is important to consider the proper ways of rescuing persons trapped in debris. This problem has been given careful attention by the Office of Civil Defense, which recommends the techniques described below.

Debris Handling

Debris should be removed with care. Since it is difficult at times to recognize a body in the midst of debris, picks should not be used unless there is no likelihood of a victim being near. Shovels and other tools also must be used carefully. Any debris close to a casualty should be removed by hand; heavy gloves will increase the efficiency of debris removal.

As debris is removed, it should be taken by wheelbarrow or basket to an area well away from the building and one where it cannot block traffic. Removed debris in piles should be marked by a sign so that other rescuers do not start sifting through it again, looking for casualties. Sound lumber may be saved to provide supports.

All workers should avoid unnecessary walking around on the debris, since this may cause additional collapse of material on top of buried casualties. As the removal of debris continues, the leader on the site should continually evaluate the likelihood of further collapse of walls, ceilings, or floors on rescuers and victims. If there seems to be any danger of this

---

* Raker, J. W. *et al. Emergency Medical Care in Disasters.* National Academy of Sciences—National Research Council, Washington, D. C., 1956, p. 21.

occurring, the remaining structure should be shored up and stabilized at once. No attempt should be made to return any part of the structure to its original position; this might only cause further collapse. The aim of shoring is the prevention of any further movement of debris.

When working in debris, extreme caution should be used in handling electric wires and gas pipes. Also, pools of water near electric wires are to be avoided. In general, the electric or gas supply to a single damaged building may be shut off by a volunteer rescuer at the master switch or shut-off valve for that building. However, large street mains and high-voltage equipment should be handled only by utility or public works maintenance crews.

Tunneling through debris to remove victims is both slow and dangerous; it should be attempted only if other methods seem to be impractical. A trained engineer should supervise such activity.

Rescue Materials

One of the most important rescue materials is rope. Rope may be used to hoist injured persons, to erect makeshift derricks, to help lift heavy debris, to make lifelines, and for other purposes. The safe working strength of rope should be known; otherwise, there is the danger of a broken rope dropping a heavy load and causing greater injury and damage. Safe working strengths of new manila rope are:

⅜ inches in diameter	270 lbs.
½ inch in diameter	530 lbs.
⅝ inches in diameter	830 lbs.
¾ inches in diameter	1,080 lbs.
1 inch in diameter	1,800 lbs.

If old rope is used, it should first be tested for strength. Wire rope is approximately eight times as strong as manila, but it is not usually available near a disaster, nor can untrained volunteers handle it properly. Nylon rope is seldom available in large enough diameters to be of use in a disaster. Rope should not be passed over sharp edges. It should be handled carefully and the knots tied properly.

Ladders are also important rescue devices. In some situations they are used to ascend or descend. However, they are useful also as temporary bridges across unstable debris, as stretchers to which injured persons can be tied securely to be raised or lowered through openings, and as legs for makeshift derricks.

A block and tackle, if available, is useful in providing a mechanical advantage in lifting heavy debris.

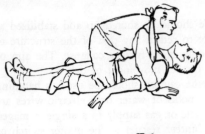

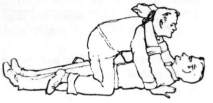

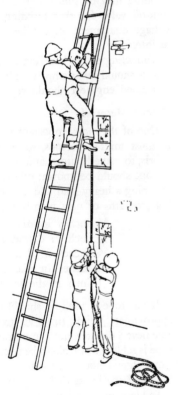

Fig. 1. Fireman's drag. Two ways of tying an unconscious casualty to the rescuer in a narrow space.

Fig. 2. Helping a person down a ladder with a safety line.

Fig. 3. Casualty lashed to stretcher.

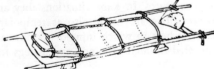

Figs. 1-6. Redrawn from Rescue Skills and Techniques, Technical Manual TM-14-1. Office of Civil Defense, Department of Defense, November, 1962.

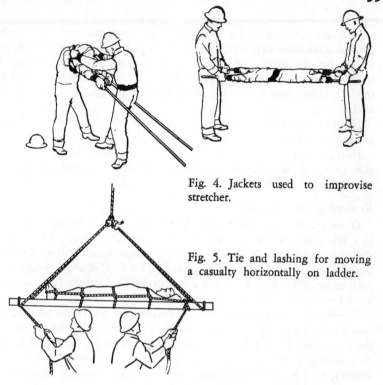

Fig. 4. Jackets used to improvise stretcher.

Fig. 5. Tie and lashing for moving a casualty horizontally on ladder.

Fig. 6. Casualty being hoisted from cave-in with tie and lashing.

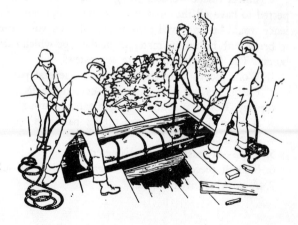

Jacks are useful in lifting extremely heavy loads but must be used by persons with some experience in this field. Jacks can be used to lift the weight but should not be used to hold the weight up, particularly if rescue workers are going to crawl under it. Once the weight is lifted by the jack, cribs, made of heavy timbers, can be put underneath to hold the load.

Hand tools of various sorts are needed to help remove debris. Included are shovels, saws, bolt-cutters, crowbars, and so forth.

Heavy rescue equipment, such as winches, cranes, blowtorches and power-saws, should only be used by persons who have had considerable experience in handling them.

Removing the Casualty

Often, the casualty may have to be removed from a damaged building to a safe place outside before first aid can be administered. Every effort should be made to select a method of movement which will do the least additional damage to his existing injuries. However, in some situations—such as an impending fire—this may not be practical, and the casualty must be removed as quickly as possible.

The fireman's drag is useful where a rescuer must remove an unconscious casualty from a cramped space. Safety lines may be used to help a rescuer carry a victim down a ladder. If the situation permits, an excellent way of removing a casualty is to lash him securely to a stretcher (or small ladder), so that the stretcher can then be carried, lowered, or raised by ropes to a place of safety (Figs. 1-6).

Volunteer Rescue Kit

Volunteer rescue workers going to the scene of a disaster cannot be expected to have all the needed tools and equipment. However, their efficiency would be improved considerably if each volunteer would remember to bring with him some materials of the type which can be found in most homes. The following items are suggested:

1. Work gloves (preferably leather)—several pairs.
2. Flashlights and extra batteries—even if the disaster took place during the day. Rescue operations might extend through the night.
3. A clean sheet (to be torn up for bandages).
4. Several clean towels.
5. Rope—at least ½" in diameter.
6. Smooth pieces of wood or metal suitable for splints.
7. A crowbar, if available.

13 FIRST AID

First aid is the initial help given to an injured person. It may be administered by a physician, nurse, policeman, soldier, scout, or anyone else.

The importance of prompt, proper first aid, unfortunately, is not fully understood by most persons. In past disasters, less than 10% of the injured were given any observable first aid before being rushed to hospitals.* Many laymen, apparently, think of first aid as being applicable mainly to minor wounds. When major injuries are encountered, they seem to feel that only a hospital can help the victim, and so make virtually no attempt to administer first aid. This is a serious error.

Generally speaking, the greater the injury, the greater the need for appropriate first aid before evacuation. This principle, somehow, must be more widely taught to the public.

Perhaps one illustration will help. Surgeons usually do not operate on patients in shock, since the added strain of surgery would probably cause death. Instead, they first use anti-shock measures of various sorts, including transfusions, to bring the patient out of shock and into a condition in which he can survive an operation. These anti-shock measures may take hours. Now, let us assume we were dealing with a victim of an accident or disaster who has a broken leg but is not in shock. Appropriate first aid (splinting) may take 15 minutes but when the patient arrives at the hospital, he will probably be in good enough condition, so that surgery can be started rather promptly. If, on the other hand, in the rush to get the patient to the hospital, splinting is neglected, about 15 minutes will be saved, but the patient is likely to develop shock as the result of being moved without a splint, and a simple fracture may become compound. On arrival at the hospital, he may need several hours of anti-shock therapy before he is ready for surgery. The 15 minutes saved by omitting first aid may result in a net delay of hours. In cases where bleeding is severe, lack of first aid may cause death.

The purposes of first aid include:

1. Maintenance of respiration.

* Bowers, W. F. and Hughes, C. W. *Surgical Philosophy in Mass Casualty Management.* Charles C. Thomas, Springfield, Ill., 1960, p. 104.

2. Stopping of bleeding.
3. Prevention of shock.
4. Prevention of further damage to soft tissues from fractured bones.
5. Protection of the wound from further contamination.
6. Relief of pain and discomfort as much as possible.

There are excellent texts on first-aid procedures and these, therefore, need not be considered here in any detail. However, it is appropriate to discuss briefly a few of the basic principles as they relate to a disaster situation.

Before starting first-aid procedures, a quick survey of the entire patient should be made, so that the most important measures are undertaken first. A sucking wound of the chest must be closed at once, even if non-sterile materials, like clothing or cardboard, have to be used temporarily. If at all possible, a doctor or nurse should give first aid to such patients. If a patient has trouble breathing because of damage to the larynx, a tracheotomy may be needed. Here, too, a doctor or nurse should perform this procedure.

Bleeding should be stopped by means of pressure bandages. Tourniquets are dangerous and should be used as a last resort only. In general, a tourniquet should be applied only if pressure bandages do not work, and if it has been decided that the limb involved will have to be amputated. For this reason it is best to have a physician assume the responsibility for applying a tourniquet.

Splinting is essential before patients with fractures are moved. No one other than a doctor should attempt to straighten a broken limb before splinting. If a broken limb is bent at the break, it should be splinted as it is. Professional splinting supplies will probably not be available for most disaster victims, so makeshift splints will have to be made from debris, etc. It would be helpful to practice such use of makeshift splints well in advance of any disaster.

Bandaging of wounds is a useful first-aid measure, which may prevent further contamination and which usually helps stop bleeding. In disasters of any size, sterile or even clean bandages in the area will probably be insufficient. Accordingly, doctors, nurses, and other medical personnel on the way to a disaster scene, may want to stop at drugstores in the support area and load up with sterile supplies. Antiseptic solutions, ointments, etc., should be avoided since they don't help, and are apt to hinder later surgical procedures.

In a civilian disaster, the medication to the injured should be administered only by a doctor or nurse, or under their direct supervision.

14 EVACUATION

Evacuation is the movement of the victims from the impact area to a safer area, or to a medical installation for more specific care. In past civilian disasters the impulse has been to evacuate the injured directly to hospitals. However, the military services have found that it is better to evacuate in stages. Initially, the injured are given first aid in the field. Then they are brought to a forward aid station where a doctor gives additional first aid, plasma if needed, and medication. A partial sorting then takes place, with the cases needing immediate surgery being sent more rapidly to the next installation. At the next point, more extensive procedures can be performed, and so on.

This sort of arrangement, while quite efficient, requires training and experience. It probably cannot be completely adapted to civilian disasters. However, a partial adaptation is practical, and could be of major benefit to disaster victims. Medical collecting points could be set up around the periphery of the impact zone, adjoining main roads. The injured, given first aid where they are, could then be carried by stretcher, or in some instances in vehicles, to the medical collecting point. Here, a doctor or nurse (or both) could check the adequacy of first-aid measures, administer medication where advisable, and even give plasma, if it is available. Following this, the injured could be loaded into vehicles and sent to hospitals. Meanwhile, a message could be sent to the hospitals, notifying them of the number of casualties to expect. This, in turn, would increase the efficiency of the hospitals.

Evacuation patterns should be planned in relation to the number and kind of casualties, and the hospital capabilities. In general, it is unwise to swamp the nearest hospital, as has been done in the past. If there are several hospitals in the area, casualties should be sent to them in proportion to their capacity. Sometimes, the nearby hospitals may not have the ability to handle all the injured. In such cases, *direct* evacuation of some of the injured from a medical collecting point to more distant hospitals would be advisable. This would avoid placing additional burdens of sorting and transshipment on the local hospitals, and would insure better, earlier, and definitive care for the casualties. As the evacuation of casualties proceeds, it will usually be found that the slightly injured reach collecting points before the seriously injured, since the former seldom have to wait for litters and similar help. If they are then evacuated quickly to the nearest hospitals, they may overload its facilities and make the job of helping the seriously injured more difficult. Accordingly, a physician or nurse, staffing a medical collecting point, should give serious consideration to evacuating the minor injuries to relatively distant hospitals.

Evacuation of casualties should be done by large vehicles (trucks and buses), whenever possible. These vehicles can carry litter patients quite comfortably, if the litters are securely lashed in place. A first-aid attendant can travel in each vehicle to make sure that splints and bandages remain in place. Furthermore, it is much easier to control evacuation patterns when large vehicles are used. An excellent choice for both ambulatory and litter patients is the school bus. Because of its distinctive color, it is readily recognized and can be routed through traffic jams with minimum delay.

In some major disasters, air evacuation should be considered for serious burn cases (see chapter 18). These patients can usually be transported by air safely for the first 24 hours; afterwards, transportation of any sort becomes more hazardous. If a large number of serious burn cases (burns of more than 20% of the total skin area) result from a disaster, these cases could be transported by air to large cities throughout the nation. This spreading of the load would greatly improve the care available to each patient, and would make available to most of them such specialized life-saving equipment as the artificial kidney. If air-evacuation of burn cases is decided on, some sort of medical collecting and treatment unit should be set up at the airport. Burn cases arriving there could receive anti-shock therapy, including oral anti-burn solution (see chapter 33), plasma, and intravenous morphine before emplaning. A doctor and/or nurse, with additional plasma and medication, could go along on the plane to insure the arrival of the patients in good condition.

Hospitals in the destination city should be notified in advance, and doctors and nurses should be sent to the airport to receive the casualties. This type of procedure can be facilitated by a long-distance telephone call to the MEND (Medical Education for National Defense) coordinator of a medical college in the destination city, who can be asked to help coordinate the efforts of the hospitals to receive, distribute and treat the incoming casualties.

15   HOSPITAL CAPABILITIES—MAJOR SURGERY

The ability of hospitals to handle disaster victims is usually exaggerated by the general public. This explains why local hospitals are generally swamped after a disaster, a condition which often results in confusion and inefficiency. In some cases in the past, poor medical care was given because of overloading. In the Texas tornado disaster of 1947, "the hospitals became very quickly a sort of madhouse, with everybody running in to see what was happening."* An estimated 5,000 sightseers clogged the hospitals.

"After the explosion and fire in Chicago, involving fewer than 85 casualties, 5 city hospitals were almost completely disrupted by the sudden influx of patients."** Note that this was only 18 casualties per hospital. In 1955, a bridge collapsed in a town of 7,000; about 30 workmen were injured. Even with evacuation of the more seriously injured to a large city 200 miles away, and the importation of surgical teams, the last patient was not operated upon until 72 hours had elapsed.***

Clearly, the experience in past disasters throughout the nation shows that the average hospital is seldom, if ever, able to handle the load of emergency cases following a moderate disaster. In part, this is due to confusion, lack of planning, and lack of realistic training for emergencies. However, it is also due to a basic lack of understanding of the capabilities of hospitals. A 200-bed hospital can handle 200 *assorted* patients who come and go in a staggered fashion, but if even 20 seriously injured patients come in at once, the hospital would be unable to handle them, unless there had been some unusual foresight, planning, and training.

Let us assume that a hospital has a good disaster plan, well-trained personnel, and that through good luck and excellent coordination with police and civil defense officers, it manages to avoid the congestion and confusion of convergence. Let us further assume that it has the facilities and equipment common to most American hospitals today. Approximately how many serious casualties could it handle, and what would be the limiting factors?

* Moore, H. E. *Tornadoes over Texas.* U. of Texas Press, Austin, 1958, p. 22.
** Lueth, H. C. Emergency Medical, Hospital, and Nursing Care. *Ann. Amer. Acad. Pol. and Soc. Sci., 309:* 142, Ja. 1957.
*** Bowers, W. F. and Hughes, C. W. *Surgical Philosophy in Mass Casualty Management.* Charles C. Thomas, Springfield, Ill., 1960, p. 96.

This information is important for anyone who may become involved in disaster management. In order to make intelligent decisions on the routing of casualties to hospitals, it would be most helpful—and often life-saving—to be able to estimate how many severe casualties could receive appropriate surgery in each hospital within a reasonable period of time.

In severe wounds, the maximum delay before surgery should not exceed six hours, but in few disasters has it been possible to accomplish this. A realistic decision should be made as to the extent of delay which can be considered acceptable when dealing with many serious casualties requiring surgery. It is suggested that the surgical experience in World War II may be a useful guide. Despite the difficulties in locating the casualties and transporting them to hospitals, approximately 70% of the severely wounded were operated on within 12 hours of being wounded—not 12 hours after admission to the hospital.* It seems reasonable, therefore, to select the 12-hour interval as the maximum delay of surgery that can be tolerated in any disaster situation where there is an option to transfer some of the casualties to another city. Aside from a thermonuclear war, or a tremendous earthquake, this option of transferring casualties to other areas is usually available.

According to World War II experience, a well-trained surgeon with ancillary personnel should be able to do seven to nine emergency, life-saving operations on severely wounded persons in a working day. The length of the working day is not specified, but it seems to be 12 hours ordinarily, and longer in emergencies. Probably, a figure of seven operations per surgical team within 12 hours is a realistic estimate for most hospitals, provided other factors do not cause delays.

The availability of operating rooms may be a limiting factor, though emergency operating rooms can sometimes be added. The ratio of operating rooms to total bed capacity varies with the type of hospital. Therefore, it is best to base casualty handling ability on the number of operating rooms, rather than on the number of beds. As a range, one may estimate that general hospitals will have one operating room for every 20 to 40 beds.

The availability of surgeons is seldom a limiting factor. Usually, there are enough surgeons to utilize all of a hospital's operating rooms continually for a 12-hour period.

* Beebe, G. W. and DeBakey, M. E. *Battle Casualties*. Charles C. Thomas, Springfield, Ill., 1952, p. 100.

Thus, the ability of a 350-bed hospital with ten operating rooms to handle seriously injured disaster victims within the stipulated 12-hour interval should approach 10 x 7, or 70, *provided no other limiting factors interfere.*

A search for additional possible limiting factors has revealed some interesting and important facts. The supply of blood and plasma for transfusions is not a limiting factor in most disasters. (It might be in thermonuclear warfare.) Usually, each hospital has an adequate reserve of plasma and blood, and long before this reserve is used up, additional blood is sent from Red Cross regional supply depots. In the past the Red Cross has not waited for requests for blood but has sent it to hospitals upon receiving the disaster report from its own local chapter, or from other sources. This extra blood supply usually arrives in less time than it would take to draw and type blood from donors at the hospital. It is true that in past disasters the use of blood and plasma to combat shock has been less than it should have been. However, this was not the result of a shortage, but was due to confusion and poor planning, which, in turn, prevented sound medical judgment.

A major limiting factor in the ability of civilian hospitals to handle severely injured disaster victims is a shortage of surgical instruments. The average civilian hospital has close to the minimum number of instruments and few reserves. If there are ten operating rooms, several are equipped and used for the surgical specialties—such as eye, ear, nose, and throat, and so forth. While the rooms themselves could readily be used for general surgery, the instruments would not be satisfactory for this purpose. Furthermore, the distribution of the seriously injured cases is usually such that most of them require general or orthopedic surgery. A general hospital with ten operating rooms is likely to have no more than five sets of instruments suitable for general or orthopedic surgery. This still does not mean that five major operations can be performed simultaneously on disaster victims, since it takes time after an operation to clean the instruments, pack them, and sterilize them. In order to use an operating room on a continuous basis, there should be at least two full sets of instruments for each operating room. While one set is in use, the other would be washed, packed, and sterilized. This need for two sets introduces an additional limiting factor.

Thus, it is estimated that the actual ability of most civilian hospitals to provide emergency major surgery for disaster victims is approximately one-quarter of the potential ability based on its number of operating rooms and surgical staff. Therefore, unless some steps are taken to obtain instruments, the ability of an average civilian hospital to provide emergency surgical care to seriously injured casualties in a 12-hour period may be estimated as: number of operating rooms x 7 x $\frac{1}{4}$. This means that the 350-bed hospital with ten operating rooms mentioned above could probably only take care of 18 of these serious casualties in one 12-hour period—even without confusion and convergence. In actuality, the capability might be reduced still further by the disorganization and confusion following a disaster.

Let us consider the steps which could be taken—and have been taken—to counteract the limitations imposed by an instrument shortage. The immediate steps which can be taken after a disaster has struck are unfortunately somewhat limited. In the Worcester tornado, the doctors in one hospital decided to overcome the instrument shortage by eliminating the sterilization procedure; they washed the instruments in tap water and then used them on the next case. As might have been predicted, the incidence of wound infection was well over 50%, and approached 100%, according to some estimates.

After the Texas City explosion, the Galveston hospitals also experienced an instrument shortage. A request was made to the Red Cross for help and the Red Cross purchased new instruments in St. Louis and Chicago and flew them to Texas in a Navy plane. However, supplies from St. Louis did not arrive until about 12 hours after the explosion, and the Chicago instruments arrived about 24 hours after the explosion. Obviously, these instruments could not improve hospital capabilities during the first 12 hours.

Attempts to borrow instruments from other hospitals are not likely to help much, since they, too, probably have no reserves. Emergency purchases from suppliers can seldom be put into use until many hours have elapsed. First, the shortage must be recognized, and this usually takes more than an hour. Then, the request has to be relayed to Red Cross headquarters, which can order the instruments by telephone without delay. However, the instruments must then be taken from stock, driven to an airport, and flown to another airport. From there, they must be driven to the hospital, often through jammed convergence traffic. Upon arrival at the hospital, they must be washed, assembled into usable sets, and sterilized. It is doubtful if all these steps can be accomplished quickly enough to make much of an improvement in a hospital's surgical capability for the critical first 12 hours. The emergency field hospitals, stockpiled through the country, would also be of no value during those first

12 hours since it takes 24 hours to unpack their instruments and put them into service. Let us now consider some possible long-term solutions to this problem of instrument shortage. One solution would be for each hospital to purchase enough instruments to enable it to function at full capacity during an emergency. Unfortunately, such instruments are expensive and only a few hospitals could afford them. Another solution would be for the government to purchase the instruments and store them in the hospitals. An agreement could be made that the extra instruments be kept in a secure place and be used only in a bona fide disaster. This sort of arrangement would be the most satisfactory, since it would increase the surgical capabilities of all our civilian hospitals severalfold at a minimal cost. A third solution would be the purchase of extra instrument sets by the Red Cross and their storage in packed sets in the Red Cross regional blood depots, ready for quick sterilization. When a disaster report is received, the instruments could be sent at once to hospitals in the area, along with the reserve blood, and without waiting for a formal request. This kind of procedure would make it possible for virtually any hospital to receive additional instruments within three hours or less.

Burns

The ability of most hospitals to care for burns is much less than their ability to care for lacerations, fractures, and other injuries. A severely burned patient requires more than twice as much surgical and nursing time as a compound fracture. Furthermore, some burn cases require for survival specialized equipment, such as the artificial kidney, which may not be available in every hospital. It may be helpful to separate the burn cases according to severity.

Burns comprising less than 20% of the body surface may be considered as roughly equivalent to abdominal wounds in terms of hospital capabilities. Not all of these burns will require immediate surgery; some can safely be deferred for more than 24 hours.

Burns comprising from 20% to 50% of the body surface pose a much more difficult problem. As a rough estimate, one may assume that a civilian hospital can handle one such burn case for every 100 beds, in addition to its load of other types of casualties. If burns are the only kinds of casualties, one may calculate the capability as being approximately one-half of the capability of handling assorted major surgical cases.

Burns comprising more than 50% of the body surface probably should not be kept in the average hospital at all. They should receive transfusions and other preliminary treatment, and be transferred within 24 hours to a large university hospital, its equivalent, or a military hospital.

Shock

Hospital capabilities in providing anti-shock treatment can be high if there is some intelligent planning and efficient carrying out of plans. Anti-shock therapy can be provided by internists, pediatricians, and psychiatrists. An experienced surgeon can supervise and assist a dozen other doctors. A team of one doctor, two nurses and ancillary personnel should be able to care for ten shock patients, provided there has been adequate planning.

In general, the ability of the average civilian hospital to provide anti-shock therapy should be considerably greater than its ability to provide major surgical care. Accordingly, hospitals can serve as medical way stations, providing anti-shock therapy for many casualties who must be transferred to other hospitals.

Psychiatric Casualties

The number of psychiatric casualties requiring the help of a psychiatrist is probably quite small immediately after a disaster. The likelihood is that this will pose no problem, and that psychiatrists may be used as general physicians.

Minor Surgery

The apparent ability of a hospital to provide minor surgical aid to disaster victims is usually much greater than its ability to provide major surgical aid. There are several reasons for this. Minor surgery takes less time, so that more can be done in the same period. In addition, it is less urgent, so that operations can be delayed with less risk. Fewer and simpler instruments are used, so that the instrument shortage problem is less serious. On the other hand, providing minor surgical care to large numbers of casualties might interfere with giving major, life-saving surgery to the more seriously injured. It is helpful here to use the concept of optimum minor surgical capability. This may be defined as the number of minor surgical procedures which can be performed in 24 hours without interfering seriously with the maximum capability of providing major surgical aid. The optimum minor surgical capability will depend on several factors. These include:

1. The total number of qualified surgeons available compared to the total number of operating rooms usable for major surgery.
2. The availability of clinic rooms, etc., suitable for minor surgery.
3. The availability of instruments and supplies.
4. The availability of nurses.
5. The general layout of the hospital, in terms of space, corridors, etc.

There will probably be a great deal of variation in the optimum minor surgical capability of different hospitals. In some cases, it may be less than the maximum major surgical capability; in other cases it may be several times greater. General estimates are not likely to be helpful. The administrator, the chief of surgery, or the director of nursing of each hospital should—as part of the disaster plan—make a realistic estimate of the optimum minor surgical capability of their institution and communicate that estimate to the local civil defense director. Such an estimate should take into account probable reduction in surgical staff, since some surgeons have appointments in several hospitals, and may do their work elsewhere in the emergency.

17   CASUALTY SORTING AND TRIAGE

Casualty sorting is based on the principle that the existing medical and nursing personnel and facilities be used to save as many lives as possible. One form of casualty sorting is known as triage. It involves the separation of the casualties into three major divisions.

The first division consists of those whose wounds are minor or who can safely tolerate a long delay before surgery.

The second division consists of those whose injuries are major, who require life-saving measures within a relatively short time, and who have an excellent chance of eventual recovery.

The third division, sometimes called the "expectant group," consists of patients whose injuries are either considered hopeless or are so severe that an inordinate amount of a surgeon's time would be required to save them. These expectant cases are not necessarily put aside to die. If they can be improved by nonsurgical methods, they may be transferred into the second group. After the surgeons finish work on the second and first divisions, they might be able to save some of the expectant group who still survive.

The principle of triage was developed in times of war and probably reached its peak during World War I, when there were floods of casualties which could not possibly be handled with existing surgical personnel and techniques. In World War II, although the principles of triage were adhered to, a smaller proportion of casualties was put into the expectant category. Surgical techniques had improved so that cases which would have been hopeless in World War I could now be saved. Furthermore, improved mobility of surgical teams made it possible to dispatch surgical aid to areas of high casualties with minimal delay.

Since World War II, there have been still further improvements in surgical techniques. As a result, the number of truly "hopeless" cases reaching the operating room alive is quite small in most kinds of disaster. The major justification for putting a patient into an "expectant" category would be that in the amount of time needed to provide him with proper surgical care, two or three others could be saved. However, there are reasons why this type of approach may not be applicable to most civilian disasters. First, there is no shortage of surgical capability for the nation as a whole, and patients can be transported by air, if necessary, to distant cities in time to receive life-saving care. Secondly, it is unlikely that the judgment of the triage officer will be based solely on the classical triage guidelines. Let us take an example of two patients: one is a 70-year old man who is moderately injured, and who would survive if he had an operation lasting one hour. The other is a seven-year old child with much more serious injuries who would require at least three hours of surgery in order to have much of a chance of survival. According to the classical triage principles, the 70-year old man would be operated on promptly, while the child would be put into the expectant group. Is it likely that the triage officer would adhere to this sort of principle?

Although triage was a useful method of providing the best available surgical care in World War I, there are serious doubts about its applicability to most civilian disasters today. A more recent suggestion is that a different plan of casualty sorting be developed; an outline of such a possible plan follows:

Division I. Minor injuries.

A. Cases to be handled in minor surgical operating rooms of hospitals.

B. Cases to receive preliminary first aid and then to be transferred. Transportation may be by bus, train, or automobile.

Division II. Patients requiring anti-shock treatment. These must be treated at once and cannot be transferred while still in shock.

Division III. Serious injuries, requiring major surgery. (Most patients in division II would move to division III when out of shock.)

A. Injuries which require the most rapid emergency surgery.

B. Injuries which can wait from six to 12 hours for surgery without serious risk, and who can receive such surgery at the hospital within the 12-hour period.

C. Injuries in which the risks of transferring are less than the risks of waiting more than 12 hours for surgery. These cases should be transferred promptly to other hospitals anywhere in the nation by the most appropriate method, including airplanes.

Division IV. Patients whose injuries are of such a nature as to require highly specialized equipment in order to have any chance of survival. These patients should be transferred by air to large university medical centers throughout the nation. Cases with more than 50% burns would fall into this category.

This type of sorting plan would be effective in disasters which did not involve the entire nation. However, if a disaster of enormous magnitude, such as a thermonuclear war, occurred, the regular triage procedure would be more appropriate.

18 HOSPITAL PLANNING FOR DISASTER

A realistic hospital disaster plan, with rehearsals for key personnel, can contribute greatly to the hospital's efficiency in a disaster. Although many hospitals have disaster plans, they vary considerably in practicality and realism. This chapter, therefore, will consider some important aspects of a hospital disaster plan. The emphasis given to certain details is based on reports of past disasters.

A. An estimate should be made by a committee, including the Chief of Surgery, Director of Nursing, and Hospital Director, of the probable capability of the hospital in handling emergency casualties of various sorts (chapters 15 and 16). This estimate should be realistic rather than optimistic. The numbers obtained in the estimate should be made known to all department heads and also to the local and state civil defense directors.

B. The next step should be the clear designation of areas to be used for disaster purposes. The ordinary space usage patterns will not be enough. The emergency room, designed for a handful of patients, can never accommodate 100 persons. Space must be made available in out-patient departments, basement areas, office areas, auditoriums, and even research wings. Every effort should be made to avoid using corridors for anything other than passageways. Areas designated to special functions should include:

1. A general casualty reception area. This should be as close to a suitable entrance as possible.

2. One or more areas for casualty sorting. These should be in locations which can be closed off from the general public, so that the doctors can work efficiently. The casualty sorting areas should be fairly close to the casualty reception areas.

3. A shock treatment area. This should be close to the casualty sorting area and not too distant from the blood bank.

4. Additional emergency operating rooms for major surgery, if these are to be utilized.

5. Minor surgery rooms.

6. Rooms to which off-duty hospital personnel, volunteering for disaster assignments, are to report. Small rooms may be used for this

purpose, since most of these persons should be assigned to jobs within 15 minutes of reporting.

7. Rooms in which volunteers, who are not hospital employees, can wait for assignments. These people occasionally can be of considerable help if they have had appropriate training, and if they are carefully supervised by hospital personnel. For example, retired nurses and military officers may come to volunteer their services.

8. An information area. This should be as far from the first five areas as possible. A secondary information area just outside the hospital would be of major value. It would enable anxious relatives to get some information about their missing loved ones without disrupting the efficient care of the casualties inside the hospital. A chaplain would be of great help in such an area.

C. The assignment of hospital employees to all entrances to regulate the flow of uninjured visitors is another important step. The inundation of corridors and lobbies by masses of people must be prevented at all costs. Most of the visitors will have legitimate reasons for trying to get in; they will be looking for missing relatives who may be injured. However, if allowed to enter en masse, they would disrupt the care given to the victims. Therefore, they must be kept out as gently and tactfully as possible, and the reasons for this decision should be explained to them. In some cases a few visitors may be allowed in and then, when they leave, others can be given their turn. Parents of small children who might be casualties should be given priority.

The guards at the doors should have instructions to allow entry of casualties, hospital personnel, and volunteers who can identify themselves as members of the nursing or medical professions or civil defense groups.

The plan should include assignment of guards even to those entrances which are normally kept locked. In the confusion of the disaster, one may be unlocked by a hospital employee, allowing a swarm of visitors to enter. This assignment of door guards is likely to be one of the most important single steps in an effective hospital disaster plan. Consideration should also be given to the possibility that a disaster may occur at night, and door guard assignments should, therefore, be made for all shifts.

Among the remaining parts of a proposed hospital disaster plan are the following, not presented in order of importance:

D. Hospital employees should be designated to run the automatic elevators during an emergency.

E. A communications plan should be set up, based on the assumption that the hospital switchboard will be virtually useless. Internal hospital communications can readily be handled if there is an internal dialing system. External communications would probably pose considerable problems. A short-wave radio transmitter would be a major asset. Also, one or more unlisted telephone lines, independent of the hospital switchboard, would help get vital outgoing calls through. Any coin telephones inside the hospital should be pre-empted for hospital business (*see* p. 50). Runners should be provided to carry messages.

F. Personnel should be assigned to disaster stations by name and title and the assignments be renewed, in writing, each year. Key positions include:

1. Chief of casualty sorting. This should be the most experienced surgeon available.

2. Chief of the shock section.

3. Supply officer. This should be an experienced nurse, if possible. This officer's primary function will be the anticipation of shortages before they occur. A purchasing agent could serve as deputy.

4. Chief of minor surgery section.

5. Chief of personnel. This officer's responsibility will be the assignment of off-duty hospital employees and volunteers to jobs.

6. Communications officer.

7. Information officer. This officer's major function would be to accumulate and list information about casualties, and to supply this information to relatives of the injured.

8. Coordination officer. This officer's function would include planning and putting into effect orderly patterns of casualty flow from reception area to sorting, to shock treatment, to operating rooms, to beds. In addition, this officer would notify the hospital director or his deputy whenever the load of incoming casualties became too great for the hospital's capabilities (*see* chapters 15 and 16) and recommend transfer of some casualties to other hospitals. Someone with a thorough knowledge of the hospital layout would be needed for this position, and it is likely that a senior nurse would be the best choice.

9. Morgue officer.

In addition, appropriate assistants to these key personnel should be assigned in the early stages of the plan.

G. Plans should be drawn up to transfer casualties that are in excess of the realistic hospital capability to other hospitals, including those in other cities.

H. Plans need to be made through the medical staff for discharging the less seriously ill patients to free hospital beds.

I. The hospital plan should consider the physiological limitations of its personnel and provide for relief shifts after the first eight to 12 hours. In some past disasters, hospitals were filled with an excess of off-duty personnel and other volunteers for the first few hours. But after about 12 to 18 hours, an acute personnel shortage developed, while the need for personnel remained high.

J. Multiple personnel assignments should be made for each position. Generally speaking, the first person to arrive on the scene takes over and later arrivals assist, take other posts, or arrange to cover a second shift.

If only one person is assigned to a key position, such as casualty sorting, there is the risk that that person may be out of town when the disaster strikes.

K. Provisions should be made for coordination with other hospitals and with civil defense.

L. Large hospitals may wish to consider providing forward echelons of doctors and nurses at the disaster scene.

M. The overall plan should be clear and concise. It should be written in such a way that each person involved understands clearly what his or her assignment is, aside from having a sound general grasp of how the total plan is supposed to function.

Bibliography

General

Bates, F. L., Fogleman, C. W., Parenton, V. J., Pittman, R. H. and Tracy, G. S. *The Social and Psychological Consequences of a Natural Disaster.* National Academy of Sciences—National Research Council, Publication 1081, Washington, D. C., 1963.

Clifford, R. A. *The Rio Grande Flood; a Comparative Study of Border Communities in Disaster.* Disaster Study Number 7. National Academy of Sciences—National Research Council, Publication 458, Washington, D. C., 1956.

Danzig, E. R., Thayer, T. W. and Galanter, L. R. *The Effects of a Rumor on a Disaster-Stricken Community.* Disaster Study Number 10. National Academy of Sciences—National Research Council, Publication 517, Washington, D. C., 1958.

Disaster. Volumes 1-4, 1947-1950.

Doherty, J. F. Inventory of Employee Skills for Disaster Control. *Industrial Security,* 6:39, 1962.

Drayer, C. Psychological Factors and Problems, Emergency and Long-Term. *Ann. Amer. Acad. Pol. and Soc. Sci.,* 309:151, 1957.

Ferrari, N. D. Rescue Service in Industry. *Industrial Security,* 6:56, 1963.

Fritz, C. E. and Mathewson, J. H. *Convergence Behavior in Disasters: A Problem in Social Control.* Disaster Study Number 9. National Academy of Sciences—National Research Council, Publication 476, Washington, D. C., 1957.

Fritz, C. E. and Williams, H. B. The Human Being in Disasters: A Research Perspective. *Ann. Amer. Acad. Pol. and Soc. Sci.,* 309:42, Ja. 1957.

Instituut voor Sociaal Onderzoek van het Nederlandse Volk. *Studies in Holland Flood Disaster in 1953.* By the Instituut and the Committee on Disaster Studies of the National Academy of Sciences—National Research Council, Washington, D. C. The Hague, 1955, 4 vols.

Killian, L. *A Study of Response to the Houston, Texas, Fireworks Explosion.* Disaster Study Number 2. National Academy of Sciences—National Research Council, Publication 391, Washington, D. C., 1956.

Lemons, H. Physical Characteristics of Disaster: Historical and Statistical Review. *Ann. Am. Acad. Pol. and Soc. Sci.,* 309:1, Ja. 1957.

Leopold, R. L. and Dillon, H. Psycho-Anatomy of a Disaster—A Long-Term Study of Post-Traumatic Neuroses in Survivors of a Marine Explosion. *Am J. Psychiatry, 119*:913, 1963.

MacMahon, B., Pugh, T. F., and Ispen, J. *Epidemiologic Methods*. Little, Brown, Boston, 1960.

Natural Disasters. Navdocks, P-88, Department of the Navy, Washington, D. C., 1961.

Perry, H. S. and Perry, S. E. *The Schoolhouse Disasters*. Disaster Study Number 11. National Academy of Sciences—National Research Council, Publication 554, Washington, D. C., 1959.

Red Cross Disaster Manual. American Red Cross, Washington, D. C., 1955.

Robinson, D. *The Face of Disaster*. Doubleday, Garden City, N. Y., 1959.

Stiles, W. W. How a Community Met Disaster: Yuba City Flood, 1955. *Ann. Amer. Acad. Pol. and Soc. Sci.*, 309:160, Dec. 1957.

Stone, J. B. Industrial Mutual Aid Associations for Emergencies. *Industrial Security* 6:89, 1962.

Taylor, I. and Knowelden, J. *Principles of Epidemiology*. Little, Brown, Boston, 1957.

Technical Manual: *Rescue Skills and Techniques*. TM-14-1, Department of Defense, U. S. Government Printing Office, Washington, D. C., June 1959.

Wallace, A. F. C. *Tornado in Worcester*. Disaster Study Number 3. National Academy of Sciences—National Research Council, Publication 392, Washington, D. C., 1956.

Wambach, A. G. Planning for Emergency Repair and Restoration. *Industrial Security* 6:98, 1962.

Wolfenstein, M. *Disaster: A Psychological Essay*. The Free Press, Glencoe, Ill., 1957.

Medical, Surgical, and Hospital

Beebe, G. W. and DeBakey, M. E. *Battle Casualties*. Charles C. Thomas, Springfield, Ill., 1952.

Blocker, V. and Blocker, T. G. The Texas City Disaster. *Am. J. Surg.*, 78:756, 1949.

Bowers, W. F. and Hughes, C. W. *Surgical Philosophy in Mass Casualty Management*. Charles C. Thomas, Springfield, Ill., 1960.

Campbell, P. E. and Jones, R. M. Experiences in the Handling of a Disaster in a Small Hospital. *Hospital Management*, 83:52, June 1957.

Churchill, E. D. Panic in Disaster. *Ann. of Surg.*, 138:935, 1953.

Coates, J. B. Jr., and Hoff, E. C. *Preventive Medicine in World War II:* Vol. 2, Environmental Hygiene. U. S. Government Printing Office, Washington, D. C., 1955.

Curry, G. J. Immediate Care and Transportation of the Injured. *Bull. Am. Coll. Surgeons*, 44:32, 1959.

Disaster Medicine: Mass Casualty Treatment Principles. *Pennsylvania Med. Journal,* 65:608 and 975, 1962.

Dunstan, E. M. Deputy Director of Hospital Civil Defense. *Hospital Management,* 83:56, June 1957.

Family Guide, Emergency Health Care. Office of Civil Defense and Public Health Service, Washington, D. C., 1961.

Freeman, L. W. First-Aid and Transportation for Patients with Spinal Cord Injuries. *J.A.M.A.,* 171:140, 1959.

Glass, A. J. Management of Mass Psychiatric Casualties. *Military Medicine,* 118:335, 1956.

Hamptom, O. P. Jr. Transportation of the Injured. *Bull. Am. Coll. Surgeons,* 45:55, 1960.

Hasenburg, H. Rehearsal for Disaster. *Hospital Management,* 86:6, July 1958.

Hill, M. E. Here's What We Learned in Treating Disaster Victims. *Hospital Management,* 79:41, Apr. 1955.

Kane, A. A. Emergency Transportation of the Injured. *N. Y. State J. Med.,* 58: 2229, 1958.

Kennedy, R. H. Disaster in Missoula. *Bull. Amer. Coll. of Surgeons,* 47:350, 1962.

Klinghoffer, M. Practical Problems in Developing Medical Plans for Disaster. *N. Y. State J. of Med.,* 63:2565, 1963.

Krueger, E. G. and Mohacsy, I. Transportation and First-Aid in Patients with Spinal Cord Injuries. *N. Y. State J. of Med.,* 59:3369, 1959.

Kulowski, J. Emergency Care of and Ambulance Organizations for Crash Victims. *Canad. Serv. Med. J.,* 11:575, 1955.

Letourneau, C. V. The Helicopter Hospital. *Hospital Management,* 89:38, March 1960.

Littleton, J. T. Moving the Acutely Injured: A Neglected "Disease." *Pennsylvania Med. Journal,* 65:1231, 1962.

McGrath, R. Doctors Need Fire Safety Training, Too. *Modern Hospital,* 99: 96, Dec. 1962.

McGrath, R. Dress Rehearsal for Disaster. *Modern Hospital,* 85:57, Aug. 1955.

McGrath, R. Rescue Procedures Can and Must Be Taught. *Hospitals; J.A.H.A.,* 30:42, Dec. 1956.

McGrath, R. Use Trucks to Transport the Injured. *Modern Hospital,* 86:70, Feb. 1956.

Saylor, L. F. and Gordon, J. E. The Medical Component of Natural Disasters. *Am. J. Med. Sci.,* 234:342, 1957.

Scheidt, A. H. Dallas Tornado Caught Them Fully Prepared. *Modern Hospital,* 88:62, May 1957.

Shaeffer, J. R. Rx for Disaster: Austerity, Simplicity, Disparity, Improvisation. *Hospital Topics,* Oct. 1962.

Spencer, J. H. And in Steelton. *Bull. Amer. Coll. of Surgeons,* 47:351, 1962.

Stout, G. N. Here's A Well Organized, Frequently Rehearsed Plan. *Hospital Management,* 80:44, Sept. 1955.

Symposium on Emergency Health Services. *Canadian Medical Association Journal,* Vol. 87, No. 22, Dec. 1, 1962.

Taft, J. A. Jr. Tornado Drill. *Hospital Management,* 89:6, March 1960.

The Victims' Reaction to Disaster. *Hospital Management,* 80:42, Sept. 1955.

Walker, R. W. Emergency Evacuation of Chronically Ill Patients. *Hospital Management,* 88:91, July 1959.

Wallace, R. E. Don't Overlook Mental Hospitals in Disaster Planning. *Hospital Management,* 85:47, Jan. 1958.

NURSING IN DISASTERS

II

In this section, some of the special aspects of nursing in disasters are considered. A special section is devoted to this area because of the critically important role of nurses in all disasters. Readers who are not nurses are invited to read this section also, in order to be better able to coordinate their own disaster role with that of the nurse.

19 THE NURSE'S ASSETS RELATING TO DISASTER

The next seven chapters are devoted to a discussion of some of the duties and responsibilities that nurses may have to assume in disasters. In such a discussion it may be helpful to point out first some of the special assets of nurses in relation to disasters. An understanding of these assets should serve to allay some of the anxiety and hesitation which most persons feel on being confronted with tasks and responsibilities of this magnitude. It is fundamentally important to recognize that no one can function perfectly in a disaster situation; the nature of disaster makes this impossible. Therefore, the standards of excellence that are used in measuring the performance of daily tasks for which there have been long periods of training and experience cannot be used to gauge performance in a disaster.

What a nurse can do in a disaster situation cannot be compared with her efficiency in her usual work. If she works in a hospital after a disaster, her efficiency may be somewhat less but her contribution will be great. If she works in the impact area after a disaster, her activities and contributions should more properly be compared to the activities and contributions of the untrained volunteers who do most of the work at disasters.

Let us first list some of the major assets which the average nurse brings to the disaster, and then let us consider how they help fit her for a major role in coping with the problem.

Some of the assets we will consider are:

1. The image of the nursing profession held by the general public.
2. The ability of the nurse to teach.
3. The ability of the nurse to lead and organize.
4. The nurse's understanding of trauma and first-aid principles.
5. The nurse's knowledge of what physicians and surgeons can accomplish in a given period of time.
6. The nurse's knowledge of contagious diseases.

In our view, the most important asset which the nurse has is the image of the nursing profession held by the average person. In ordinary times, the nurse is liked, respected and looked up to because of her contributions to mankind. She is also considered a leading expert in health problems who is particularly adept at practical, effective solutions. Because of this image, she is in an excellent position to teach the importance of disaster prevention. The teaching might be formal, through talks to PTA's and other groups, or it might be informal, during daily conversations. As is pointed out elsewhere in this book, disaster prevention is the most valuable contribution which can be made.

When a disaster actually strikes, the usual high regard for the nurse takes on an even greater depth and intensity. The nurse (and the physician) then become symbols of great significance. When people see death and destruction all around them, the fundamental importance of human life and health comes to the foreground; the preoccupations, possessions, and status symbols of ordinary days lose much of their significance. Psychological guidelines are disrupted. In this confused and frightening situation, the survivor of a disaster sees the nurse and the physician not only as helpers, but also as symbols of professions which have always placed human life and health above other considerations.

Onlookers and volunteers, to a lesser but still important extent, share in this attitude. For this reason, it is easy for a doctor or a nurse to assume a position of leadership in a disaster situation, provided that their identity as doctor or nurse is known. (Other professions such as dentistry, sanitary engineering, veterinary medicine, and laboratory technology also are devoted to the same general goals of preserving human life and health as medicine and nursing are. However, the general public is less aware of their contributions and less likely to regard them as important symbols in a disaster.)

The ability of the nurse to teach develops from her daily contacts with patients in which she teaches them various things. This ability can be utilized in teaching principles of disaster prevention, formally or informally. It may also be used in teaching first aid and emergency procedures to volunteers interested in developing such skills.

The ability of the nurse to lead and organize is often not fully appreciated. Nurses are the actual and effective leaders of most hospital personnel. The entire organizational pattern of a hospital ward or unit is based on the nursing service. Furthermore, the hospital nurse is accustomed to maintaining a smoothly functioning organization in the face of all sorts of disruptions and emergencies. She sees to it that one patient is admitted to the ward, while another is sent to surgery and another to radiology, meanwhile she administers medications, charts records, works with the physician, and so forth. The pattern changes every day, and yet order and efficiency are maintained. With this background of experience, the nurse is highly qualified to organize or help organize the various efforts to assist disaster victims.

The nurse's understanding of trauma and first aid can be an important asset in planning and conducting rescue, first aid, and evacuation procedures.

The nurse's knowledge of what physicians and surgeons can accomplish in a given period of time can be of great value in helping to plan the distribution of injured persons to hospitals.

The nurse's knowledge of contagious diseases is a major asset in handling the later stages of disasters. She can help prevent secondary epidemics by teaching, planning, inspecting, immunizing, and so forth.

It seems clear that a person with the assets discussed above could be a most valuable contributor to all phases of disaster prevention and relief. It is hoped that a clearer understanding of these factors will encourage those who may not be sure of their ability to help in the next disaster.

20 NURSING SPECIALTIES AND DISASTER

Since nursing is fairly well specialized, nurses in different positions will bring various skills to a disaster scene. This is often not recognized outside the nursing profession and is a fact that should be better understood. The principle of utilizing persons in functions most closely associated with their daily work holds true for nursing, too. This point, while seemingly obvious, has been difficult to get across.

Most people assume every nurse knows how to do everything in nursing. This simply is not true. Nursing has become as specialized a profession as any other. The technical skills of nursing are lost if not used. The ability to relearn may remain high with most nurses, but relearning takes time. In addition, there have been many changes in nursing in the past 20 years.

The public attitude of expecting a nurse to remain fully proficient in her profession, even after years away from it, probably increases the insecurity felt by the inactive nurse. Refresher courses for inactive nurses should be an ongoing part of the local disaster planning of any community. If these courses were available, inactive nurses might be able to keep up with their profession and feel more secure about their ability to help.

Both the American Nursing Association and the National League for Nursing are organized according to nursing specialties. (Their exact functional categories need not concern us here.) The American Nurses Association, through its local districts, attempts to maintain an up-to-date file of all nurses living within a geographic area. (It is an important part of disaster planning to know where all the nurses live.) This is a fairly efficient method of keeping track of actively employed nurses who are members of the ANA, but it is less efficient in the case of inactive nurses and non-members of the association.

For the purpose of disaster needs, nurses may be classified as hospital nurses, and non-hospital nurses.

Each nurse should decide for herself where her talents could best be utilized, and what added training she might need to keep ready for her role in time of community need.

But we should also realize that circumstances may make it advisable for a nurse to function in an area outside of her specialty. The same is true also of the medical profession. Medical disaster plans call for psychiatrists to give blood transfusions, and pediatricians and internists to help the surgeons, should a disaster strike and a shortage of doctors develop.

In an acute nurse shortage, nurses may have to handle situations for which they feel inadequately trained. A shift in responsibility of this nature is likely to provoke feelings of inadequacy and insecurity. These may be markedly lessened by prior training in disaster management. It would also be helpful to keep in mind the fact that nobody functions perfectly in a disaster. One must do one's best and accept the fact that one's performance will probably fall short of normal expectations.

The fundamentals of disaster nursing do not belong to any particular nursing specialty but are the domain of the entire nursing profession. The most effective role for a particular nurse in a disaster may depend on her nursing specialty; on the other hand, it may also be determined by her location at the moment of impact. For example, an operating-room nurse would obviously be extremely valuable following her specialty in the hospital after a disaster. However, if she happened to be within a few blocks of the impact area, she might contribute even more by helping to organize rescue, first-aid and evacuation efforts at the scene. Later, as others arrive at the impact area, she may decide that the needs of the situation have changed, and that she can contribute more by returning to her hospital to work in surgery. The decision as to where she is most needed at any particular moment has to be made by her. At the same time, she should realize that here, too, she may not make the best possible choice. In the confusion immediately after the impact, it may take hours before the extent of the disaster is recognized and the nursing specialist will therefore have to decide how she can best contribute to the overall effort of helping the disaster victims. A clear understanding of the phenomena attending disasters, as well as of her own specialty, will help her choose the best course of action.

Many inactive nurses are mothers. In a disaster, a mother's first thoughts will be for her own family. Nurses who are mothers should plan first to satisfy their family's needs and then to assist the disaster preparedness plan of the community. This secondary role could be in either of the major categories: hospital or non-hospital nurses.

21 NON-HOSPITAL NURSES IN DISASTERS

Non-hospital nurses generally include the following:
Public health nurses: visiting nurses, county nurses, consulting nurses, school nurses, occupational health nurses.
Nursing educators.
All other nursing specialties.
Office nurses.

A major role for all public health nurses and nursing educators is that of leadership in disaster prevention and education activities. All nurses should help teach the public the principles of disaster prevention and casualty care. Logically, the leadership for this undertaking should come from the public health nurse and the nursing educator.

During the threat, warning, and impact stages, the public health nurses should be able to utilize their knowledge of the health inventory of a defined area. The value of a plan of action by public health nurses can hardly be overestimated. Confusion and loss of precious time will prevent a maximum contribution unless there are well thought out plans.

Public health nurses should know some of the inactive nurses in the community and call upon them to assist. These inactive nurses, most often homemakers, sometimes volunteer their services in the community on health councils, PTA's, and usually are at least casually aware of health needs. The inactive nurse has definite limitations, and we must remain aware of them. However, her limitations are far less serious than the limitations of the untrained volunteer who provides most of the help in the impact area.

The school nurse may be described as a specialized public health nurse. Her help in a disaster will be most effective within a school system. The school nurse should work closely with the school administration in an effort to define all phases of a disaster plan. To draw up an evacuation scheme is the first step toward such a plan.

An essential part of keeping children safe in a time of disaster is the decision when to send them home. Time, distance, and mode of transportation should weigh heavily in this decision. Usually, the school principal and/or superintendent should make this decision and base it on his acquaintance with the geography of the area. The school nurse should work closely with each class- or home-room teacher on special situations in which she previously may have been involved. Examples of such situations include a working mother not at home during the day, and children without proper clothing.

Most schools have well defined fire evacuation plans with regularly held drills. As pointed out in chapter 36, there is often room for improvement. It is likely that if a school does not have fire drills, it will not have a school nurse either. This situation may be found in small, rural schools. A county nurse then might undertake to educate the community on the needs for fire safety.

The school nurse, knowing the facilities of the school, should also preplan the use of the building as a temporary housing point for victims evacuated from their homes. School buildings are commonly and logically used for this purpose in times of hurricanes, floods, and other disasters. The maintenance of sanitary living conditions, principally in the areas of eating and toileting, will be essential. The hot lunch program in schools is often managed by on-the-job trained women and may or may not be under the supervision of a dietitian. The food workers may need to rely on the nurse for guidance in a disaster situation. The janitorial staff may similarly need assistance in handling problems of waste disposal. The nurse may be the only trained person available to guide sanitary mass feeding and waste disposal in a school.

The school building might also be used as an immunization or first-aid center. The school health office, which is already set up, would be a logical location for this emergency service. The nurse may make arrangements in advance for volunteer assistants. She should also estimate the additional supplies which might be needed and have a plan for obtaining them from the nearest source of supply.

If a school building were ever involved in violent, sudden destruction at a time when all the occupants (teachers and children) are inside, the school nurse may be the only health-trained individual available who could improvise a plan of action quickly. Previous military training, studies of past disasters, and experience in leadership would all be of great value in such a situation.

If a school nurse is not needed in her own defined area after a disaster, she might be able to report to the impact area or to a nearby hospital. She should determine where she could be most helpful, taking into account her skills, her training, as well as the probable needs of the situation.

A public health nurse normally deals less with acute illness than with planning for the total care of the patient, and with follow-up long-term care in all its facets. Her specialties, therefore, are less the technical aspects of care as they are the sociological and psychological aspects of health. Accordingly, in a disaster situation, the public health nurse might make her maximum contribution by organizing the crowd around the impact area and helping bring order out of chaos. She might assist victims, their neighbors, and the general community during the inventory phase by lending the stability needed to minimize dazed, random behavior.

The help which a nurse can provide at the impact site is multiplied many times if she is readily identified as a nurse by her uniform. If there isn't time to put on a complete uniform, the nurse's cap is a familiar symbol which will identify her as a person to whom other rescue workers can turn for direction, advice, and guidance.

If public health nurses are not needed in the impact area, they might report to a hospital and help take charge of the relatives of the victims. The importance of having a health-trained person manage the victims' relatives has been emphasized by every nurse who has ever lived through a real disaster. If a chaplain is not available, the nurse may have to assume the spiritual duties which are often required at this time of great emotional crisis.

If, in a nuclear attack, psychiatrists are needed for general medical functions, public health nurses may assume their role—a recommendation which has been put forth by the American Medical Association.*

Public health nurses will assume responsibility for the care of many disaster victims during the recovery phase. Reconstruction of the human body can seldom be totally achieved, but rehabilitation can. It is here, in the aftermath of disaster, that the public health nurse will make her major contribution. It will be slow; it will receive relatively little notice; and, it may extend over years.

The occupational health or industrial nurse may also be described as a specialized nurse. She may or may not be more accustomed to trauma in her daily functioning than other public health nurses. Her efforts in a disaster, as those of other nurses, should be exerted in an area where most use could be made of her talents. An industrial nurse could be important within a plant in helping to organize and train a rescue and/or first-aid team of volunteers which would serve within the geographic area of the plant.

Nursing educators are classified as non-hospital nurses. However, many a teacher of nursing at present is still associated with a hospital. Her most important skills—training and organizing—will be in great demand both

* AMA *Report on National Emergency Medical Care*. Chicago, 1959.

at the disaster site and at the hospital. In an actual disaster, she will have to decide how she can best contribute to the over-all goal of minimizing loss of life, disability, and suffering, and act accordingly. Most likely, she will contribute more by organizing and directing students and ancillary personnel than by attempting to help the victims herself.

22 HOSPITAL NURSING SERVICE DURING A DISASTER

The effectiveness of the hospital nurse during a disaster will be in direct relation to the preplanning by the hospital administration. The nursing service division should participate actively in such planning. Little or no planning may result in a waste of the nurses' time and effort, and disaster victims may receive poor or little care in a disorganized and confused fashion. Well conceived disaster plans, reviewed, revised, and rehearsed, will result in rapid and effective hospital care.

The nursing service is the largest department in any hospital. It is the department that holds the hospital together 24 hours a day, but at the same time it is dependent upon the hospital administration to define its responsibility. This is necessary for day to day functioning, and is essential in disaster planning. The form that this definition of responsibility takes will determine whether the nurse will be able to function in her most important role. Lack of adequate plans could force nurses to perform supportive non-nursing functions which could be handled by other hospital personnel with lesser degrees of training and experience.

At the same time, it is also possible that the nurse may have to function in a medical assistant role if the medical staff, under the direction of the hospital administration, has not drawn up clear-cut disaster plans.

Disasters do not occur in an orderly fashion nor do they always occur when the hospital is well-staffed by the medical and administrative groups. But the nursing service is always there. Consequently, it is very likely that a disaster, happening after 5:00 P.M. or on a holiday or a weekend, will be managed during the first hour or two—or perhaps longer—with the leadership of the nursing service.

There are 168 hours in a week. Administrative and other offices are open approximately 40 hours a week, minus holidays. This leaves 128 hours, or 76% of the week, during which the nursing service department may be called upon to take decisive action on urgent problems which, during the other 24% of the time, are handled by other departments.

In the larger hospitals there are often assistant hospital administrators routinely scheduled to take care of management problems that arise after the general office hours of 5:00 P.M. If this position were occupied by someone with experience in medicine or military service, he might be in a position to manage the early hours of disaster involving a hospital. If his background does not include military, medical, or previous disaster experience, he might find it advisable to turn over the disaster management to the nursing supervisor, until an appropriately trained administrator or member of the medical staff can reach the hospital.

Possibilities such as these should be taken into account by the hospital administration and/or the committee on disaster when management plans for this contingency are formulated.

23 HOSPITAL NURSES DURING HOSPITAL FIRES

Hospitals are potentially among the most dangerous buildings in modern society. Combustible and explosive materials are stored in substantial quantities; oxygen is available under pressure and is in use 24 hours a day. The ratio of ablebodied to disabled persons is lower than in most other areas. Hospital personnel become accustomed to using dangerous equipment and, working in an atmosphere of high human tension, and may lose sight of the hazards around them. Carelessness on the part of hospital personnel may develop unless there is an ongoing and active disaster prevention program.

It has been observed that people with lower educational and training backgrounds are being employed more and more frequently as aides in hospital nursing services. The nursing shortage will not be discussed in this book; however, we must not lose sight of the fact that hospitals must take this shortage of professional nurses into account when disaster plans are formulated. It cannot be ignored.

The first and most important role of the hospital nurse is to prevent disasters from happening. Because the nurse is there 24 hours a day, she falls heir to the policeman's role and should be the key to prevention as well as to planning. At every hour of the day and night she must be alert to the danger of fire. When nursing rounds are made, the slightest smell of smoke should be investigated promptly.

Nurses often find fire doors propped open to improve ventilation or to facilitate passage. These fire doors must remain closed if they are to function when needed.

Nurses must constantly be alert to visitors and patients who smoke near oxygen. Even the medical staff, sad to say, all too often smoke near patients who are receiving oxygen. This, aside from the danger, sets a poor example to the subordinate hospital staff. The nurse as the coordinator between the medical and hospital staffs should have the courage and tact to correct the physician who has careless smoking habits.

Nurses must prevent late-hour smoking in bed by patients, and see that ether and other inflammable materials used in patient care are not left in some forgotten drawer of a treatment room without the proper safety measures.

Crowded conditions in hospitals can prevent rapid evacuation in time of disaster. Examples include beds in halls, and three beds in a room where floor space and the law allow two or one. These conditions are all too common in hospitals. Factors which create such crowding must be corrected if hospitals are to give safe care.

On the other hand, nurses must avoid alarming ill patients unnecessarily by their efforts to teach disaster prevention.

Even though waste disposal, housekeeping, closets, and so forth are not usually the direct responsibility of the nurse, after 4:30 P.M. the nurse must be alert to these areas as potential fire hazards.

A written fire prevention plan is essential for a hospital. A general organization plan should be available on which terms and titles are defined, and the plan should be so designed that it meets the specific needs of the hospital. The staffing plan of all hospital departments should be considered when the general plan of organization is defined.

The following points should be included in a fire prevention plan:

1. Reporting of fire. The need for immediate reporting of all fires, even small ones, must be emphasized. The smell or appearance of smoke must also be reported immediately.

2. Chain of command in a hospital disaster.

3. Exit routes.

4. Alternative exit routes, depending on location of the fire.

5. Availability of chemical extinguishers and training in their use.

6. Availability of water supply for fire hoses.

7. Responsibility for patient evacuation. Nursing services will need physical assistance which can be predetermined.

8. Identification of areas to which patients will be evacuated.

9. Need for equipment to give continuing care.

10. Need for continuous training of all personnel, on a scheduled basis, in fire prevention, fire fighting, and patient evacuation. The course originated by Robert McGrath is an excellent example.*

Fire drills, held regularly and observed by firemen, are of great value. The drills will impress all hospital personnel with the importance of fire safety.

The nursing department, because of its 24-hour presence in the hospital, should assume a leadership role in fire prevention.

* McGrath, R., Fire and Helpless People. *Canadian Nurse*, 53: 904, Oct. 1957.

24 HOSPITAL NURSING CARE OF DISASTER VICTIMS

A hospital nursing staff that knows how to function should a disaster strike the hospital, will be in the best position to know what to do if victims of a disaster elsewhere are brought to the hospital for care.

City and/or county planning for proper utilization of hospital facilities for disaster victims is essential. In past disasters it has happened that a few hospitals were flooded with victims while others, a short distance away, had few casualties to care for. Clearly, this type of imbalance must be avoided, and sound planning is necessary to utilize hospital facilities in the most effective manner. The city disaster plan should be known and understood not only by nurses and doctors but also by local police, ambulance drivers, funeral directors, taxicab companies, schools, volunteer groups, and so forth.

Members of the medical and nursing staffs should know their disaster posts and duties. These two groups will usually be given transportation priorities by the police. If advance arrangements are made, they may be able to receive similar priorities from taxicab companies.

If a disaster occurs late in the evening or on a weekend it would probably be advisable for all hospital nurses to report to their own hospitals immediately, since staffs are short at these times. In rare instances a nurse may report to a hospital nearer her home to give assistance. In most instances nurses employed in hospitals will be most useful at the hospital. A possible exception would be a nurse who happens to be in or near the disaster area at the time of impact.

A hospital should have close enough contact with the police and fire departments so that it can be notified in advance to expected casualties. A 15- to 30-minute advance notice to the hospital administration, division of nursing, or superior in charge of nursing could make the difference between efficient care and chaos.

Within these 15 or 30 minutes a communications plan can go into effect and hospital employees can be notified by a predefined chain system to return to the hospital. This communications plan can be handled by each department separately or by the personnel department, depending on the size of the hospital and the community. It should not be handled through the hospital switchboard, but through its pay phones. A pyramid plan should be worked out by which one person outside the hospital who has been called, telephones two or three others before reporting for duty. Thus, few of the calls need to be made from hospital telephones.

Personnel should be taught not to call their hospital in time of disaster. They should be instructed to return to the hospital as soon as possible and report to their posts on hearing of a disaster from any source. This might cause some minor hardships since so many married nurses have children, and may necessitate a pooling of children in one home with a sitter.

Entrances should be manned by hospital employees who know the plan and the employees well, and who are strong enough, physically, to keep unauthorized people out. Men from the business and personnel offices would be suitable; nursing personnel, generally speaking, should not be utilized for this purpose. However, since it is important to secure the entrances as soon as possible, it may be necessary in the early stages to use orderlies as door guards until the other personnel arrive. This is so essential that it must not be overlooked or underestimated.

One of us (E.E.) has had some first-hand experience with this kind of problem. In Des Moines, Iowa, in 1959 a young disturbed boy flew an airplane wildly over the city for four hours, terrorizing the entire city. He crashed outside the city about 4:40 in the afternoon and was brought to Broadlawns Hospital. The press and curiosity seekers so invaded the emergency room of that hospital that it was impossible to give the boy proper care. And in this instance only one victim was involved! As pointed out in other chapters, similar problems have arisen in other hospitals throughout the country after disasters.

The physical structure of a hospital will determine its plan of action and its initial screening and tagging areas. Most hospitals have an emergency room; some have clinics directly adjacent to it. All hospitals have linen rooms and cafeterias, and most have auditoriums, conference rooms, or waiting rooms. These and other similar spaces may be utilized for the initial sorting of victims. Supplies such as fluids, blood, bandages, splints, medications, and so forth can be brought there. Emergency kits can be ready in central supply, and additional packs can be prepared during the 15- to 30-minute warning period.

Medical care teams should consist of doctors, nurses, clerks, and messengers. The doctor diagnoses and prescribes care; the nurse works with the doctor in the rendering of care; the clerk writes the patient's name, diagnosis and prescription on a tag and attaches it to the patient; the messenger assists the teams, fetches supplies, delivers messages, and helps to move patients to another area for continual care, or to one assigned for their discharge home.

Cots can be temporarily used for the victims. If cots are not available, the injured can be placed on mats, blankets, or even on the floors.

While these teams are in action at the hospital emergency facilities, other teams can be screening the regular hospitalized patients for possible early discharge. This may be advisable in order to free hospital beds for some of the victims. However, the doctor in charge of the patient is the person who must make the final decision on whether he or she can be discharged early. In order to make such a decision wisely, he will need the opinion and advice of the nurses who have been caring for that patient. Accordingly, they should be prepared to make recommendations to the doctor as to which patients might be considered for early discharge.

Space should be provided for anxious relatives waiting for news, a measure which has proved to be highly important. This undertaking should be supervised by competent nurses who understand the total disaster plan of the hospital. These nurses will be able to reassure the relatives and thus assist in the smooth functioning of the disaster plan.

By keeping friends and relatives from wandering around the hospital and getting in the way, the nurses assigned to this task may increase the efficiency of doctors and nurses considerably. On the other hand, it is advisable to be prepared to handle hostile attitudes from waiting relatives and friends. They may ask why a nurse should be with them instead of caring for the seriously injured. A truthful, but discreetly phrased, answer should be prepared in advance. Psychiatric nurses might be the logical persons to handle this task and chaplains, if available, can give invaluable assistance.

Let us now consider the time (described in chapter 22) when the average hospital is administered directly by the nursing service department. Obviously, the nursing department should assume a major role in developing a disaster plan for the hours (about 128 per week) when it constitutes the overwhelming majority of all skilled and professional personnel actually in the hospital. The nursing department may have to direct virtually all functioning for the first hour or two, until staff doctors can arrive. Hospital administrators or assistants who are not trained or experienced in disaster management would be wise to relinquish their daily "boss" role and allow the nursing department to assume the major leadership role for this interval. Internes may start giving advanced first aid and treatment for shock, but for overall management of the problems they should look to the nurse for guidance, since internes usually stay in a hospital only one year and cannot be expected to know all the intricacies of its workings.

If a hospital has a residency program, the residents may be able to assume the leadership role, if they have had some previous training in the care of mass casualties. The senior resident might then share the leadership with the senior nurse present until the staff doctors arrive.

Upon receiving word of an emergency, the nurse in charge should appraise the situation and take the following steps:

1. Estimate staff available: nursing, housekeeping, and maintenance.

2. Estimate the number of critical patients already in the hospital who still require intensive care.

3. Divide the available nursing personnel into two groups, and assign as follows:

  a) one group to remain with the hospital patients,

  b) one group to report to the emergency area.

4. Activate plans to assign returning nursing personnel to the regular patients or to the disaster area. The proportions would vary, depending on the type and number of regular patients and the magnitude of the disaster.

5. Orderlies may be sent to secure entrances. When relieved, orderlies would report back to the nursing office for further assignments.

6. Activate plans to secure and distribute supplies properly.

7. Place additional patient carts and wheel chairs near emergency area.

8. Set up and staff an area for relatives of the victims.

Constant reappraisal of the total situation will be necessary. Adjustment and flexibility will be necessary as the situation changes.

25 NURSING PERFORMANCE IN DISASTERS

A review of several specific disasters illustrates the important part nurses have had in providing prompt, effective care to the injured. The interdependency of all groups, both professional and lay, is demonstrated along with the major leadership role played by nurses.

An emergency exemplifying good disaster management is the Indianapolis Coliseum gas explosion.* On October 31, 1963, shortly after 11:00 P.M., a gas explosion ripped through the coliseum, killing 68 persons and flooding Indianapolis hospitals with 385 blast victims. All the local hospitals performed well in handling the emergency.

The entire community shouldered the burden of caring for the injured. At the scene, volunteers worked side by side with policemen, firemen, doctors, and nurses. The injured were transported to local hospitals in cars, station wagons, and trucks.

Local garages sent wreckers to lift heavy pieces of concrete from trapped victims. Construction companies sent large cranes to handle debris beyond the capacity of the wreckers. Without being called, physicians, nurses, and other health personnel reported for duty both at the scene and at the hospitals.

Conventioners attending the meeting of the American Federation of Licensed Practical Nurses reported to local hospitals for duty. Student nurses provided invaluable aid in preparing supplies, answering telephones, and staffing rest areas for anxious relatives waiting for news.

Many donors appeared at hospital blood banks and Red Cross stations, and by early morning no further blood was needed.

To maintain security, the Methodist Hospital, which received the largest number of casualties (120), locked its doors, posted guards at them and in the parking lots, and barricaded all drives. Relatives of the injured were sent to a building behind the hospital where coffee, doughnuts, and news about the injured were available.

A disaster critique held five days after the explosion suggested the following areas needing refinement in future planning:

* How Indianapolis Hospitals Met Blast Emergency. Special Report. *Hospitals*, 37: 17, 1963.

1. Hospitals were not notified promptly of the disaster.

2. Proper distribution of patients to hospitals could not be made because rescue workers at the scene could not communicate with the hospitals.

In spite of the early lack of communication, the hospitals of Indianapolis demonstrated a high degree of competence in meeting this crisis. No hospital reported any shortage of personnel. This undoubtedly played an important part in the rapid, effective care given to victims despite limited early communication. By early morning, all hospitals were back to more or less normal functioning.

It should be noted that the disaster involved a relatively modest number of casualties in relation to the resources of the city of Indianapolis. If a disaster of similar magnitude had taken place in a town of 50,000, or if more people had been injured in Indianapolis, the problems might have been much more difficult to solve.

In the evening of June 20, 1957, a tornado hit Fargo, North Dakota, a city of 59,000 persons. Casualties might have been in the thousands had it not been for the weather bureau and a group of radio and television newscasters. Timely warnings allowed many people to reach shelter. Nevertheless, 150 were injured and needed care.

St. Luke's Hospital (200 beds) became a disaster relief center because of its close location to the major area of destruction, and a report of its experience is illuminating.* Shortly after the tornado hit, the hospital experienced a temporary blackout, but electricity was soon restored by emergency generators and vital sections of the hospital were supplied with power. Had it not been for this emergency generator, disaster operations would have been almost impossible.

Employees of the hospital reported back to work even though many of them had just had their homes damaged or completely destroyed. Personnel working at the time the tornado struck remained at their posts.

On the night of the tornado, the hospital had been filled to capacity. Patients who could be, were discharged; single rooms were made into double units.

One of the largest areas of responsibility fell to the nursing services. This included the coordination of emergency centers with the in-patient sections, and the overseeing of the central dressing room and the housekeeping department. Although the disaster struck when the hospital was minimally staffed, off-duty nurses returned at once, and volunteer nurses from other outlying towns reported to help.

* Short, P. L. It Did Happen Here. *Amer. J. Nursing, 59*: 228, 1959.

Rescue operations in the impact area were begun immediately. Rescue workers searched by flashlight and car headlights, looking for the dead and injured. Through wind and rain, patients were brought to the hospital on doors, improvised carriers, and stretchers. Vehicles had difficulty passing through littered streets containing convergers. Fallen electrical wires provided an element of danger.

As the patients arrived at the hospital, it soon became apparent that the facilities in the emergency receiving unit had to be expanded. The housekeeping department, under instructions from nursing supervisors, created a temporary receiving unit in the hospital cafeteria. Mattresses were placed on the dining tables and floors, and the record room personnel tagged the patients. Groups of doctors and nurses organized into teams which checked all patients. They treated and released those with minor injuries, and admitted the others either to the nursing units or directly to the operating area. The operating area involved all four suites throughout the night.

The absence of confusion was accounted for in large part by the early organization of nurses, waiting to receive the injured. Within four hours, the main load of patients had received preliminary care.

The hospital disaster committee reviewed the experience and made the following recommendations for improvement:

1. The hospital should provide as permanent equipment a patient tag to include name, address, injury, medication given, and religion.

2. Canvas stretchers should be available for use in sorting. Extra sheets and blankets, and small portable oxygen tanks would also be helpful.

3. A team of nurses should be assigned to the sorting area with the primary assignment of cleansing wounds.

4. A shock ward should be provided.

5. Areas should be provided for waiting relatives and friends to prevent crowding of halls and treatment centers.

6. A central dispatch desk should be set up, so that nurses could be assigned to the area of greatest need and then reassigned as needed.

A third example of interest took place in Canada.* At about 2:15 P.M., October 25, 1960, an explosion occurred in a chain store in Windsor, Ontario. The impact area was about three-quarters of a mile from Grace Hospital, a Salvation Army hospital, and about 70 casualties were admitted to that institution. A physician who had prepared the hospital disaster plan, happened to see the explosion from his office and telephoned the

---

* John, E., Preparedness Pays. *Canadian Nurse,* 57: 369, 1961.

hospital at once. Thus, this hospital had the advantage of prompt notification and utilized it effectively.

The assistant director of the nursing service, who was in the hospital, organized nursing and other personnel to handle the expected casualties. Operating room nurses prepared areas outside the operating theaters where chairs and beds were to be placed for patients awaiting surgery. One nurse was given full responsibility for narcotics; graduate and student nurses were sent to assigned positions to prepare to receive casualties. The switchboard was alerted to contact doctors and ask them to report to the hospital immediately.

Head nurses of various areas arranged for discharge of patients who could safely be sent home. The accounting personnel were organized for the identification of patients, and their transportation within the hospital. By the time the first ambulance arrived, 20 minutes after the explosion, the hospital was organized and ready to receive the casualties.

The nursing office also served as the information center. Extra nursing personnel were needed for the first night. There was a minimum of confusion throughout the entire proceedings.

This disaster clearly proved the value of a realistic plan and of prompt notification.

It is hoped that other nurses who participate in disaster work will write up their experiences for publication. Identification of imperfect areas in planning and performance would help others to improve their own functioning. At the same time, positive identification of areas that functioned efficiently is helpful in showing what can be done.

Bibliography

Allen, G. F. Five Hours to Zero. *Nursing Outlook,* 5:417, 1957.

A.N.A. Convention Report 1962: What to do in Emergencies. *Am. J. of Nursing,* 62:96, 1962.

A.N.A. Special Committee on Nursing in National Defense: Nursing in Disasters. *Am. J. of Nursing,* 60:1130-1133, 1960.

A.N.A. Sponsors Conference on Disaster Nursing. *Am. J. of Nursing,* 56:781, 1956.

Babcock, C. A Place for Old Folks to Live. *Hospital Management,* 85:47, Feb. 1958.

Barnett, F. R. *Women's Role in National Defense.* Yearbook of Mod. Nursing, 1959, Putnam, New York, p. 5.

Brantl, V. M. and Brown, B. J. Operation Rebound. *Am. J. of Nursing* 58: 1550, 1958.

Campbell, P. and Jones, R. M. Experiences in the Handling of a Disaster in a Small Hospital. *Hospital Management,* 83:52, June 1957.

Campion, F. Women to the Rescue. *Canadian Nurse,* 51:95, Feb. 1955.

Carlisle, B. Would Your Hospital Be Prepared? *Hospital Management,* 80:39, Sept. 1955.

Cleveland, L., King, T. and Olson, M. Disaster Day. *Am. J. of Nursing,* 56:464, 1956.

Committee on Disaster Planning, American Hospital Assoc.: Principles of Disaster Planning for Hospitals. *Am. J. of Nursing,* 56:1046, 1956.

Committee on Disaster Studies: Emergency Medical Care in Disasters, A Summary of Recorded Experiences. *Am. J. of Nursing,* 57:1200, 1957.

Committee on Disaster Studies: Social Aspects of Wartime Evacuation of American Cities and the Child and His Family in Disaster. *Am. J. of Nursing,* 57:91, 1957.

Dennis, C. L. Disaster and its Aftermath. *Am. J. of Nursing,* 61:74, 1961.

Denton, F. H. Police and Firemen Help Prepare Students for Disaster Nursing. *Nursing Outlook,* 9:28, 1961.

Derby, A. C. Early Medical Management of Mass Trauma. *Canadian Nurse,* 53:389, May 1957.

During the California Floods. *Am. J. of Nursing,* 56:439, 1956.

Earthquake. *Nursing Outlook,* 12:57, May 1964.

Fisk, H. L. and Herr, J. W. Nurse Assistants in Civil Defense. *Nursing Outlook,* 2:362, 1954.

Gardiner, L. A. Public Health Nursing in Time of Disaster. *Am. J. of Nursing,* 58:861, 1958.

Gerds, G. Without Warning. *Am. J. of Nursing,* 60:984, 1960.

Hasenburg, H. Rehearsal for Disaster. *Hospital Management,* 86:6, July 1958.

Henrietta, Sr. M. Nurses Star in Disaster Test. *Nursing Outlook*, 5:414, 1957.

Hill, E. Here's What We Learned in Treating Disaster Victims. *Hospital Management*, 79:41, Apr. 1955.

Howell, L. N. A Statewide Disaster Training Program. *Nursing Outlook* 5: 144, 1957.

Hurricane Audrey and the Red Cross. *Am. J. of Nursing*, 57:1289, 1957.

Johnson, E. Preparedness Pays. *Canadian Nurse*, 57:369, Apr. 1961.

Journal Staff: Remove the Patient, Fight the Fire, Start Evacuation. *Am. J. of Nursing*, 57:766, 1957.

Kinch, A. Bellevue Responds When Disaster Strikes in New York City. *Am. J. of Nursing*, 59:504, 1959.

Learning to Prepare for Disaster. *Am. J. of Nursing*, 60:515, 1960.

Linden, M. C. Some Psychological Aspects of Rescue Breathing. *Am. J. of Nursing*, 60:971, 1960.

Lueth, H. C. Emergency Medical, Hospital, and Nursing Care. *Ann. Amer. Acad. Pol. and Soc. Sci.*, 309:142, Jan. 1957.

Lueth, H. C. Meeting Disaster, *Am. J. of Nursing*, 56:1135, 1956.

MacGregor, J. E. In Time of Need. *Canadian Nurse*, 52:517, 1956.

Magnussen, A. K. and Schafer, M. K. Nursing in Disaster. *Am. J. of Nursing*, 56:1290, 1956.

McArthur, A. C. Nursing Care of Psychiatric Casualties. *Canadian Nurse*, 53: 456, May 1957.

McGrath, R. Fire and Helpless People. *Canadian Nurse*, 53:904, Oct. 1957.

Meehan, M. R. What the Con Edison Power Failure Did to Us. *Hospital Management*, 89:72, Apr. 1960.

Nabbe, F. C. Community Preparation for Disaster. *Am. J. of Nursing*, 55:62, 1955.

Nabbe, F. C. *Disaster Nursing*. Littlefield Adams, Patterson, N. J., 1961.

Neal, M. Hawaii Disaster. *Am. J. of Nursing*, 55:1074, 1955.

Neal, S. E. Civil Defense is Now. *Am. J. of Nursing*, 60:1303, 1960.

N.L.N.: Nursing During Disaster: A Guide for Instructors in Basic Professional Programs and Practical Nurse Programs (1951) and 1954 Supplement. *Am. J. of Nursing*, 55:1121, 1955.

Nursing Service for Disaster. Yearbook of Mod. Nursing, 1957-58, Putnam, New York, p. 223.

Nursing Service in Disaster. Yearbook of Mod. Nursing, 1959, Putnam, New York, p. 179.

Owens, E. and Schaefer, M. Volunteers in Emergency Medical Service. *Am. J. of Nursing*, 55:1248, 1955.

Packaged Hospital. *Am. J. of Nursing*, 57: 1443, 1957.

Palmer, R. T. Emergency Evacuation and Exit Drill. *Hospital Management*, 89:48, March 1960.

Peterson, A. Report from the Committee on Nursing in National Defense. *Am. J. of Nursing,* 57:604, 1957.

Piercey, W. D. and Fryer, G. E. Hospital Preparedness. *Canadian Nurse,* 53: 386, 1957.

Poole, D. Preparing Hospital Nursing Staffs for Disaster Service. *Nursing Outlook,* 6:586, 1958.

Psychological First Aid in Disasters. *Am. J. of Nursing,* 55:437, 1955.

Rayner, J. F. How Do Nurses Behave in Disaster? *Nursing Outlook,* 6:572, 1958.

Reeson, I. Nursing Care of Traumatic Injuries. *Canadian Nurse,* 53:395, 1957.

Ridgway, J. M. The Nurse in Disaster Medical and Health Programs. *Nursing Outlook,* 5:41, 1957.

Ross, J. P. Building a Hospital Disaster Plan. *Am. J. of Nursing,* 57:1461, 1957.

Sargent, A. A. It's Time for Hospitals to Lead. *Hospital Management,* 89: 40, March 1960.

Schafer, M. K. *Nursing Programs for Disaster and Defense.* Yearbook of Mod. Nursing, 1956, Putnam, New York, p. 291.

Seidlinger, E. One Way to Get Heat During an Emergency. *Hospital Management,* 77:118, May 1954.

Sharkey, G. Red Cross Nurses in the Texas Flood. *Am. J. of Nursing,* 55:310, 1955.

Sheldon, N. S. Bibliography on Nursing in Defense and Disaster. *Am. J. of Nursing,* 55:1352, 1955.

Short, P. L. It Did Happen Here. *Am. J. of Nursing,* 59:228, 1959.

Sloane, A. Disaster Nursing in the Curriculum. *Nursing Outlook,* 5:75, 1957.

Spitz, N. K. Preparing Students for Disaster Nursing. *Nursing Outlook,* 4: 149, 1956.

Staff: How Blackwell's Plan Provided Relief to Victims. *Hospital Management,* 80:46, Sept. 1955.

Stewart, A. C. Ready to Serve. *Am. J. of Nursing,* 63:85, 1963.

Stout, G. N. Here's a Well-Organized, Frequently Rehearsed Plan. *Hospital Management,* 80:44, Sept. 1955.

Taft, J. A., Jr. Tornado Drill. *Hospital Management,* 89:6, March 1960.

The National League for Nursing and National Defense. *Nursing Outlook,* 7:233, 1959.

To Morocco on a Disaster Nursing Mission. *Am. J. of Nursing,* 60:357, 1960.

Tyhurst, J. S. Psychological and Social Aspects of Community Disasters. *Canadian Nurse,* 53:423, May 1957.

Virginia Association Cosponsors Conference on Disaster Nursing. *Am. J. of Nursing,* 57:222, 1957.

Virginia State Department of Health: Instructor's Manual of Practical Nursing in Disaster. *Am. J. of Nursing,* 60:874, 1960.

Walker, R. W. Emergency Evacuation of Chronically Ill Patients. *Hospital Management,* 88:91, July 1959.

Wallace, R. E. Don't Overlook Mental Hospitals in Disaster Planning. *Hospital Management,* 85:47, Jan. 1958.

When the Doria Went Down. *Am. J. of Nursing,* 56:1288, 1956.

Witt, B. E. When the Rivers Rose in Kentucky. *Nursing Outlook,* 5:420, 1957.

Zampella, A. D. General Preparedness Plan for your Hospital in Event of Emergency, *Am. J. of Nursing,* 56:1048, 1956.

MAJOR TYPES OF DISASTER

In this section, the major types of non-military disaster are considered according to a uniform set of subheadings. Through this approach, the similarities and differences in the various disasters are brought into clearer focus. The subheadings used are:

General description
Frequency and area of occurrence
Important past examples: U. S. A. and other areas
Causes
Possible preventive measures
Measures for minimizing casualties from initial impact
Recognition and warning signs
Main mechanisms of death and injury
Prevention of further casualties after initial impact
Special procedures and problems in rescue, first aid, evacuation, and definitive medical and nursing care

The important past examples are not intended as a complete listing of all disasters in the category. Some disasters in distant parts of the world have never been adequately reported. In general, it was felt that a small to moderate disaster occurring in recent years was of greater interest and importance at this time than one which occurred a long time ago. Therefore, some of the smaller disasters of many years ago have been omitted. The large disasters of the past have been listed, as well as some smaller ones which are of special interest for one reason or another.

Where the disaster lists seemed unduly long, only the most recent ones are usually included. In some cases, the listing begins after World War I, in other cases, after World War II, and in still other cases at an arbitrarily chosen date. The reader may compare any two lists by taking this into consideration. In this fashion, a fairly accurate estimate can be made of the relative tolls of different kinds of disasters.

chapter

26

AIRPLANE CRASHES

General Description

An airplane crash involves a sudden collision with another object or the earth, resulting in partial or complete destruction of the plane. Usually, the passengers are killed. We will not consider military planes.

Frequency and Area of Occurrence

Airplane crashes take place in all nations and over inhabited as well as uninhabited territory. The frequency of major crashes (those with more than 25 dead) has been approximately two per year for American planes, and slightly more for planes of other nations. This represents the greater number of American planes, rather than any increased vulnerability.

Important Past Examples—U.S. Planes, after World War II

Date	Approximate Location	Deaths
May 30, 1947	Fort Deposit, Maryland	53
June 13, 1947	Leesburg, Virginia	50
October 24, 1947	Bryce Canyon, Utah	52
November 1, 1949	Washington, D. C.	55
June 24, 1950	Lake Michigan	58
August 31, 1950	Cairo, Egypt	55
June 30, 1951	Rocky Mountain Park, Colorado	50
August 24, 1951	Decoto, California	50
December 16, 1951	Elizabeth, New Jersey	30
February 11, 1952	Elizabeth, New Jersey	33
April 11, 1952	San Juan, Puerto Rico	52
April 30, 1952	Brazil	50
February 14, 1953	Gulf of Mexico	46
July 12, 1953	Wake Island	58
October 6, 1955	Laramie, Wyoming	66
November 1, 1955	Longmont, Colorado	44
June 30, 1956	Grand Canyon, Arizona	128
April 21, 1958	Las Vegas, Nevada	49
February 3, 1959	East River, New York City	65
June 26, 1959	Milan, Italy	68
January 6, 1960	Bolivia, North Carolina	34
January 19, 1960	Holdcraft, Virginia	50

109

Date	Approx. Location	Deaths
March 17, 1960	Tell City, Indiana	63
September 19, 1960	Guam	78
October 4, 1960	Boston, Massachusetts	62
December 16, 1960	New York City	134
September 1, 1961	Hinsdale, Illinois	78
September 10, 1961	Shannon, Ireland	83
September 17, 1961	Chicago, Illinois	37
November 8, 1961	Richmond, Virginia	77
March 1, 1962	New York City	95
March 16, 1962	Western Pacific	107
May 22, 1962	Centerville, Iowa	45
November 30, 1962	New York City	25
February 12, 1963	Everglades, Florida	43
December 8, 1963	Elkton, Maryland	81
February 25, 1964	Lake Pontchartrain, Louisiana	58
March 1, 1964	Tahoe, California	85

Planes of Other Nations, after January 1, 1956

Date	Nationality	Approx. Location	Deaths
February 18, 1956	British	Malta	50
February 20, 1956	French	Cairo, Egypt	52
June 20, 1956	Venezuelan	Asbury Park, New Jersey	74
December 9, 1956	Canadian	British Colombia	62
July 16, 1957	Dutch	New Guinea	56
August 11, 1957	Canadian	Quebec, Canada	79
December 8, 1957	Argentinian	Bolivar, Argentina	62
May 18, 1958	Belgian	Casablanca, Morocco	65
June 2, 1958	Mexican	Guadalajara, Mexico	45
August 14, 1958	Dutch	Atlantic Ocean	99
October 17, 1958	Russian	Kanosh, Russia	75
September 24, 1959	French	Bordeaux, France	53
December 8, 1959	Colombian	Cartagena, Colombia	46

Date	Nationality	Approx. Location	Deaths
January 19, 1960	Unknown	Ankara, Turkey	41
January 21, 1960	Colombian	Montego Bay, Jamaica	37
February 5, 1960	Bolivian	Cochabamba, Bolivia	59
February 25, 1960	Brazilian and U.S.	Rio de Janeiro, Brazil	61
February 26, 1960	Italian	Shannon, Ireland	27
March 19, 1960	Unknown	Bogota, Colombia	38
April 22, 1960	Belgian	Congo, Africa	35
June 11, 1960	Australian	Pacific Ocean	29
June 24, 1960	Brazilian	Atlantic Ocean	51
August 29, 1960	French	Dakar, Fr. W. Africa	55
January 3, 1961	Finnish	Helsinki, Finland	25
February 15, 1961	Belgian	Berg, Belgium	73
March 28, 1961	Czechoslovakian	Ruesselbach, W. Germany	52
May 10, 1961	French	Sahara Desert	79
May 30, 1961	Venezuelan	Lisbon, Portugal	62
July 12, 1961	Czechoslovakian	Casablanca, Morocco	72
July 19, 1961	Argentinian	Azul, Brazil	67
August 10, 1961	British	Coast of Norway	34
September 12, 1961	French	Rabat, Morocco	77
October 7, 1961	British	French Pyrenées	37
November 2, 1961	Brazilian	Recife, Brazil	49
November 23, 1961	Argentinian	Sao Paulo, Brazil	52
December 22, 1961	British	Ankara, Turkey	27
March 4, 1962	British	Dovala, Cameroon	111
June 3, 1962	French	Paris, France	130
November 26, 1962	Brazilian	Sao Paulo, Brazil	23
November 27, 1962	Brazilian	Lima, Peru	97
November 30, 1963	Canadian	Montreal, Canada	118
February 21, 1964	Philippine	Mindanao, Philippines	31
February 27, 1964	Japanese	Oita, Japan	19
February 29, 1964	British	Innsbruck, Austria	83

Causes

Some plane crashes are caused by faulty design, construction, or maintenance of the plane; some result from storms; some are caused by errors in judgment on the part of the operating personnel. One crash was caused by a bomb. The cause of some crashes has never been determined.

Possible Preventive Measures

The safety of a particular plane design is a highly technical matter which seems to be adequately handled. Unfortunately, some design defects have shown up only in high-speed flight. As soon as these defects are recognized, they are usually corrected in other planes of the same type.

Scheduled airlines apparently maintain their planes properly. It is not clear whether the unscheduled lines do also.

It may be helpful to scrutinize the use of medications by flying airlines personnel. Apparently, certain types of drugs are widely used by airplane passengers and may be used by some flying personnel to prevent airsickness. Many of these drugs also have tranquillizing effects. Tranquillizing drugs tend to make the user accident prone by removing or depressing the normal and helpful anxiety which results from a potentially dangerous situation. Thus, a necessary corrective action might be delayed or omitted, resulting in a crash.

Measures for Minimizing Casualties from Initial Impact

It might be possible to design planes so that the passengers survive ordinary crashes. This would require some means of preventing fires from igniting the fuel. This field deserves considerable study and research in view of the increasing air travel.

Recognition and Warning Signs

These are usually technical and are noted by the pilots but seldom by the general public.

Main Mechanisms of Death and Injury

Abrupt deceleration on impact with the ground tears loose vital organs, or results in being crushed against plane components. If there are any survivors of the impact, they are probably killed by the burning fuel which engulfs the plane.

Prevention of Further Casualties after Initial Impact

Usually there are no further casualties after the initial impact and fire, since all concerned are dead.

Special Procedures and Problems in Rescue, First Aid, Evacuation, and Definitive Medical and Nursing Care

Usually all or most victims of airplane crashes are killed before any help can be given.

chapter

27 AVALANCHES

General Description

An avalanche is a sudden fall of a large mass of snow, ice, rock or earth from a high elevation to a lower one. Sometimes, terms like rock-slide or land-slide are used.

Frequency and Area of Occurrence

Minor avalanches occur quite often. Major avalanches, killing 50 or more persons, take place less than once a year. The areas involved are steep mountain slopes throughout the world.

Important Past Examples—U.S.A.: none reported

Other Areas, after World War II

Date	Approximate Location	Deaths
September 18, 1948	Northern Assam, India	500
February 15, 1949	Sondondo, Peru	70
January 4, 1951	Andes, Peru	132
January 22, 1951	Alps of Austria and Italy	222
July 12, 1954	Medellin, Colombia	140
February 13, 1956	Macedonia (Greece)	58
March 3, 1956	South Korea	100
January 12, 1958	Pachaco, Peru	100
June 7, 1958	Northeast India	52
January 23, 1960	Manila, Philippines	40
May 27, 1960	Rupanco, Chile	113
March 30, 1961	Moscow, Russia	145
June 30, 1961	Tokyo, Japan	80
July 5, 1961	Kerala, India	73
January 10, 1962	Ranrahirca, Peru	3,500
August 12, 1963	Nepal	150

Causes

Most avalanches result when heavy layers of snow and ice on a mountain side become warmed by the sun and slip from their former anchorage.

It is believed that when a mass of snow and ice is delicately balanced, a sudden loud noise may precipitate an avalanche. The correctness of this belief has not, however, been tested scientifically.

Other avalanches have taken place when a mass of rock suddenly split off the mountain and fell. Such an occurrence is the result of millions of years of water freezing and thawing in the cracks of the rocks.

Possible Preventive Measures

Avalanches of snow and ice can be changed from disaster to controlled, relatively safe incidents by using high explosives to blast loose dangerous accumulations of snow and ice. Before such blasting, all persons in the valleys below must be evacuated. The blasting could be done by mountaineers or by bombing planes.

Recognition and Warning Signs

People living in avalanche-prone areas generally recognize the growing danger of the accumulating snow and ice. Unfortunately, however, they don't take protective action often enough. Warning that an avalanche is on its way consists of a roaring sound, but the time available for protective action is usually too short to be effective.

Main Mechanisms of Death and Injury

Victims are crushed and smothered.

Prevention of Further Casualties after Initial Impact

The avalanche usually destroys water and sewage systems, so that action must be taken to prevent epidemics among the survivors.

Special Procedures and Problems in Rescue, First Aid, Evacuation, and Definitive Medical and Nursing Care

There are few injured survivors of an avalanche. Most victims are either killed or uninjured. Thus, there are no special problems or procedures to consider.

chapter

28   BUILDING COLLAPSES

General Description

The term "building collapse" as used in this chapter refers to the sudden falling of all or part of a building in the absence of any major outside force; the destruction of buildings by earthquake, tornado, or explosion and so forth is not included. The term "building" includes grandstands, railway stations, and other structures.

Frequency and Area of Occurrence

Building collapses are relatively infrequent in the United States and probably will vanish completely if proper building codes are maintained. Generally, old buildings are the ones that collapse. In other parts of the world, however, relatively new structures have collapsed with loss of life.

Important Past Examples—U.S.A.

Date	Place	Deaths
August 22, 1891	New York City	64
June 9, 1893	Washington, D. C.	22
January 28, 1922	Washington, D. C.	98
July 4, 1925	Boston, Massachusetts	44

Other Areas, after World War II

August 12, 1954	Palace of Lama in Tibet	700
January 25, 1959	Motion picture theater in Turkey	35
September 16, 1959	Apartment building in Italy	55
February 2, 1963	Parochial school in Ecuador	105
May 28, 1963	Railroad station in Portugal	48
January 15, 1964	Paris building under construction	15

Causes

Building collapses may be due to poor design, to badly mixed concrete,

115

or to the decay and weakening of wooden timbers. At times, overloading of an old building may cause collapse.

Possible Preventive Measures

New building codes include safety factors which should make collapse extremely unlikely. Another important preventive would be the enactment of state laws, requiring strict periodic safety inspections of all buildings over 30 years old which may contain more than 20 people, even for a short time.

Measures for Minimizing Casualties from Initial Impact

None are known.

Recognition and Warning Signs

The appearance of cracks in the outer walls may be a warning of impending collapse.

Main Mechanisms of Death and Injury

Most of the deaths and injuries are caused by crushing.

Prevention of Further Casualties after Initial Impact

The most important measure is prevention of fire.

Special Procedures and Problems in Rescue, First Aid, Evacuation, and Definitive Medical and Nursing Care

The major problem is rescue of the survivors from the debris. This involves the principles discussed in chapter 12.

29 DAM COLLAPSES

General Description

A dam collapse results in the sudden release of large amounts of water which sweep over low-lying villages, causing many deaths and injuries. Some dams are made of concrete, some of masonry, some of earth, and some of a combination of different materials.

Frequency and Area of Occurrence

Dams collapse somewhere in the world about once every year or two. Earth dams seem to be somewhat more likely to collapse than concrete dams.

Important Past Examples—U.S.A.

Date	Place	Deaths
May 31, 1889	Johnstown, Pennsylvania	2,200
March 13, 1928	Santa Paula, California	450
December 14, 1963	Los Angeles, California	3*

Other Areas, after World War II

October, 1957	Northeast India	400
January, 1959	Vega de Tera, Spain	144
December, 1959	Malpasset, France	421
March, 1960	Ores, Brazil	1,000
March, 1961	Kiev, Russia	145
July, 1961	Central Korea	250
April, 1963	Quebrada la Chapa, Colombia	50
October, 1963	Vaiont, Italy	3,000

* Fortunately, an alert inspector noticed a crack in the dam around 11 A.M. and most residents fled before the actual break occurred several hours later. Had the break happened at night, the death toll would have been many hundreds of people. This illustrates the great value of timely warning.

Causes

Dams may collapse because of a shifting of their foundation after an earthquake. They may break because of faulty construction or of oil drilling nearby. Earth dams are most likely to collapse when excessive rainfall fills the reservoir to overflowing. The excess water then pours over the top of the dam, gradually washing and cutting deep channels into it. This weakens the entire structure so that it then gives way entirely. The Vaiont dam in Italy broke when an avalanche fell into the reservoir, suddenly raising the water level far above the top of the dam.

Possible Preventive Measures

Concrete dams tend to be safer than earth dams because they are not weakened by heavy rains. An important preventive measure is the provision of large channels for releasing impounded water rapidly. When heavy rains are expected, the water level behind the dam may be lowered appreciably by opening the appropriate valves. This would reduce the load pressing against the dam. It might cause some downstream flooding, but not of a magnitude sufficient to cause fatalities.

Measures for Minimizing Casualties from Initial Impact

The basic measure for minimizing casualties is the evacuation of towns and villages below the dam before the break. Some warning signs may be available and it may be possible to develop others (*see* below).

Recognition and Warning Signs

A warning sign of a dangerous condition in an earth dam is a rise in the water level of the reservoir almost to the top of the dam. This usually follows heavy rains upstream of the dam. In general, if the rate of water level rise is such that it may reach the top of the dam within six hours, it would be prudent to evacuate all people who would be in the path of the flood waters should the dam actually give way. If the rising water actually begins to spill over the top of the earth dam, the situation may be considered much more dangerous.

Another type of warning device might be incorporated into new and existing dams of all kinds of construction. Strain gauges, attached to steel beams, could be imbedded in key locations of the dam and arranged so as to measure small displacements in three dimensions. The wires from the strain gauges would run to electronic devices in a control room. Any excess displacement of the dam would be registered in the control room and set off an alarm. Exceedingly sensitive strain gauges have been designed which can measure displacements of fractions of a millimeter.

Such gauges, some smaller than a postage stamp, measure the displacement of railroad rails under the weight of the train. By the appropriate arrangement, these gauges could distinguish displacements due to heat and cold from those stresses which might cause the dam to collapse. The use of such devices may make it possible to obtain warning of an impending dam collapse in time to evacuate all persons in the danger area.

Main Mechanisms of Death and Injury

Most casualties are caused by crushing injuries and drowning.

Prevention of Further Casualties after Initial Impact

The prevention of fire in the destroyed villages is an important measure. After the collapse of the Johnstown, Pennsylvania, dam, a large secondary fire killed many trapped victims.

Special Procedures and Problems in Rescue, First Aid, Evacuation, and Definitive Medical and Nursing Care

After a dam collapse, people below the dam are usually either killed quickly or escape without any major injuries. There are relatively few survivors requiring hospitalization.

30 EARTHQUAKES

General Description

An earthquake is a sudden slipping or displacement of a portion of the earth's crust, accompanied and followed by a series of vibrations. The slipping or displacement of the crust occurs along fault lines, i.e., lines where there are weaknesses. The actual movement is usually much smaller than is popularly imagined. The earth may only move a few feet in a severe earthquake; the damage is caused by the vibrations which are set up by the sudden movement.

Frequency and Area of Occurrence

Earthquakes occur virtually every day somewhere on the earth's crust. However, most are too small to be noticed by human senses and are identified only by special instruments. The major earthquakes occur at irregular intervals. Although earthquakes have, in the past, been concentrated in certain areas, any place on earth may be subjected to a severe earthquake at any time. Indeed, if an area has been free of earthquakes for a long period of time, there is the possibility that if an earthquake does strike, it will be a major disaster. The recent quake at Skoplje, Yugoslavia is an example.

The time of occurrence of earthquakes may be an important factor in the death toll. School buildings and certain types of commercial structures are particularly dangerous. Ordinary frame houses appear to be less dangerous. Therefore, an earthquake during school hours would be much more tragic than one at other times. The recent Alaska earthquake took place at a time when the schools and commercial buildings were closed, and many people were in automobiles on the streets. This probably accounted for the relatively low death rate.

Important Past Examples—U.S.A.

Date	Place	Deaths
December 16, 1811	New Madrid, Missouri	Not recorded

(Note: This earthquake was of major proportions by any standards. The shocks were felt distinctly as far away as Washington, D. C. There were very few people in Missouri at that time, so the casualties were low. How-

ever, if an earthquake of similar magnitude were to occur in the same general
area today, the death rate would be extremely high.)

Date	Place	Deaths
April 18, 1906	San Francisco, California	452
March 10, 1933	Long Beach, California	120
August 17, 1959	Hebgen Lake, Montana	28
March 27, 1964	Alaska	114

Other Areas

January 24, 1556	China	830,000
October 11, 1737	Calcutta, India	300,000
November 1, 1755	Lisbon, Portugal	60,000
December 28, 1908	Messina, Italy	75,000
December 16, 1920	Kansu, China	180,000
September 1, 1923	Tokyo, Japan	140,000
December 26, 1932	Kansu, China	70,000
May 31, 1935	Quetta, India	60,000
December 27, 1939	Erzingan, Turkey	23,000
September 9-12, 1954	Algeria	1,600
November 4, 1956	Iran	2,350
July 2, 1957	Iran	2,500
July 28, 1957	Mexico City, Mexico	56
December 13, 1957	Iran	1,400
December 13, 1957	Outer Mongolia	1,200
January 15, 1958	Peru	128
August 16-21, 1958	Iran	191
February 29, 1960	Agadir, Morocco	12,000
May 21-30, 1960	Chile	5,700
September 1, 1962	Iran	12,000
July 26, 1963	Skoplje, Yugoslavia	3,000
January 18, 1964	Paiho, Taiwan	110

Causes

Earthquakes are believed to result from the gradual changes in weight
distribution of the earth's crust. This sets up enormous strains and stresses

on the rock layers, and when the strain exceeds the strength of the rock, is suddenly fractures or slips along a pre-existing fault. This causes a series of shock waves which travel outward at speeds of several miles per second. These shock waves can shake certain types of building materials to-and-fro rapidly, so that they collapse.

Possible Preventive Measures

None are known.

Measures for Minimizing Casualties from Initial Impact

The major measure for minimizing casualties is better construction of buildings, so that they can resist the sudden shock waves. This does not mean heavier construction, or a marked increase in cost. It is largely a matter of design. Many modern buildings in Japan are made to resist earthquakes. The basic principle in earthquake-resistant construction is fastening the parts of the building together, so that in any sudden displacement the entire building moves as a unit and doesn't break up. In addition, certain changes in foundation plans may be needed.

Most American buildings are not earthquake resistant. Among the most vulnerable buildings are modern schools. A relatively small earthquake would collapse most of them, killing and injuring the children inside. A moderate earthquake hit Long Beach, California, on March 10, 1933. A school was completely demolished. Fortunately, the earthquake occurred at 6:00 P.M. Had it struck a few hours earlier, it would have killed hundreds of school children.

Training and education may also help reduce casualties. Those who are able to dive under a sturdy table at the first shock have a better chance of survival.

Recognition and Warning Signs

In a few cases, there have been minor tremors of the earth shortly before the main quake. However, this is not a reliable warning sign. The major quake may occur with no warning at all.

Main Mechanisms of Death and Injury

Most deaths and injuries come from collapsing buildings. People who are in open fields would probably survive a class XII earthquake (the maximum force). In some cases, people inside buildings are killed or injured when the roof falls in on them. In other cases, people running into the streets are killed when walls and roofs of adjoining buildings fall sideways into the street.

There are some misconceptions in this area. The belief that vast chasms open up in the earth, swallowing whole villages, and then closing, is without any basis in fact. Actually, the chasms and rents that do appear in the earth's surface are rather shallow and narrow. It is doubtful if, out of more than a million killed in earthquakes, as many as a dozen have died from falling into chasms.

Prevention of Further Casualties after Initial Impact

The most important measure is prevention of fire. Collapsed houses present large masses of inflammable materials. Broken gas mains and high-tension wires will add to the problem. Water mains are destroyed, adding to the fire-fighting problem. In the past, fires have caused many added deaths and much added destruction after earthquakes. In 1906, an earthquake shook San Francisco, and started fires which then produced *20 times* as much damage as the quake itself.

In 1923, after an earthquake hit Tokyo and Yokohama, fires started, and these fires killed an *additional* 100,000 people!

The possibility of a second earthquake soon after the first cannot be overlooked. Therefore, rescuers should be warned to be cautious in going into or near any buildings which are still standing.

Tsunamis (chapter 46) can cause greater loss of life than the original earthquake, and prompt, thorough warning and evacuation of low-lying areas within several miles of the coast is important. This applies to all areas less than 100 feet above sea level on the same ocean basin, even up to many thousands of miles away.

Epidemics may also be a problem after earthquakes, due to broken water and sewage mains. Early attention should be given to disease prevention.

Special Procedures and Problems in Rescue, First Aid, Evacuation, and Definitive Medical and Nursing Care

Many of the survivors injured in the earthquake area will be buried under debris. In rescuing them, care and training will be needed to prevent further collapse of masonry and timbers. Therefore, use of proper and tested methods of shoring up the debris is of great importance.

In many cases, it may be necessary to give first aid to victims who are still partially trapped.

The number of injured in an earthquake is likely to be much greater than the number injured in most other disasters. Also, local hospitals will probably be destroyed or incapacitated. Accordingly, plans should be made either to evacuate victims to other cities, or to bring in surgical teams and hospitals, or both.

31 EPIDEMICS

General Description

The medical and nursing literature on epidemics is extensive. The condensed material in this chapter merely presents a brief introduction to selected aspects, in order to emphasize some basic approaches to epidemics as disasters. For further details one of the comprehensive texts on public health should be consulted.

Epidemics are outbreaks of disease causing the sickness of large numbers of people in a short time. Epidemics have, in the past, been the greatest disasters of all. Although our present public health measures have managed to control most of them, the possibility of their recurrence must always be considered. The magnitude of epidemics seems to be unclear to most persons. For example, one hears a great deal about the tragedy of World War I. Without minimizing the tragedy of all wars, it should be pointed out that the greatest tragedy between the years 1910-1920 was not World War I, but the influenza epidemic of 1919. The total killed on both sides in World War I was about 8.5 million people; the number that died of influenza in 1919 was about 20 million. The number of American dead in World War I was about 116,000; the number of Americans who died of influenza in 1919 was over 500,000. This comparison is offered not to minimize the disastrous nature of war, but to point out the magnitude of the danger of epidemics. The fact that for a short period in human history epidemics in one part of the world have been brought under control is no guarantee that they may not recur. Furthermore, our current medical armamentarium is not sufficiently equipped to save the victims of all epidemics. It is true that we now have medications which will save the lives of most people with such dreaded diseases of the past as cholera, bubonic plague, and typhus fever. However, we still do not have any specific treatment for virus diseases like influenza. Furthermore, there have in the past been terrible epidemics which came and went suddenly, without leaving any clue to their etiology. An example of this is the "English Sweating Sickness" of 1485, 1507, 1518, 1529, and 1551. These epidemics killed about half the population of many towns.

In the history of the human race, epidemics have been by far the greatest of all disasters. Even today, the chances are that a return of some of the more malignant epidemics of the past would be no less disastrous than a thermonuclear war.

An important feature of the worst epidemics has been the susceptibility of populations which had never before encountered the disease. Some examples may illustrate this point. Measles is now considered a relatively mild childhood disease in Europe and the United States. However, when measles was first brought to the American continent, it killed many more Indians than did the weapons of the invaders. In 1531, hundreds of thousands of Mexican Indians died of measles. In 1875, measles killed 40,000 persons in the Fiji Islands, out of a population of 150,000.

The European population was, in turn, susceptible to diseases of the other areas. Syphilis was apparently a fairly mild, endemic disease in the Americas. However, when syphilis was brought back to Europe by the explorers, it developed into an epidemic disease of major severity, killing most of its victims in a period of a month or so and accounting for hundreds of thousands or millions of deaths. As the European population became partially adapted to it, its severity decreased, although it is still a major disease by any standards.

Between 1801 and 1803, the French army in Haiti had 22,000 deaths from yellow fever, out of a total of 25,000 troops.

Despite our advances in sanitation and medical and nursing care, we are extremely vulnerable to any new infectious agent that might be introduced. Some scientists have indicated that this constitutes a major risk in our space exploration program. It is quite possible that on some other celestial bodies, such as the moon and especially Mars, forms of microscopic life exist, or have evolved, which are resistant to the sterilizing agents generally available on earth, including ultraviolet rays. They point out that the most deadly material known—botulinus toxin—is produced from an organism which, in spore form, can survive hours of exposure to boiling water and later multiply, producing a deadly toxin. The virus of hepatitis also can survive long periods of boiling. Some bacterial forms live in hot water, others in sulfur springs. It is feared that somewhere on the moon, or on one of the planets, there may be microscopic spores which, if brought to earth on a returning space vehicle, might multiply and decimate or even wipe out the human race. Such fears have been expressed by recognized independent scientists but are apparently not being taken seriously by our space agency.

Of particular significance is a study conducted at Brooks Air Force Base.* An environment was produced which, to the best of our knowl-

* U.S.A.F. *Studies with a Simulated Martian Environment; Bacterial Survival and Soil Moisture Content.* School of Aerospace Medicine, Brooks Air Force Base, Texas, November 1962.

edge, was the same as that on the surface of Mars. The factors regulated were atmospheric composition (hardly any oxygen), atmospheric pressure, moisture, temperature, and soil type. Into this simulated Martian environment were introduced cultures of a test bacterium. At the end of 60 days, researchers not only found that the bacteria were alive, but that they had multiplied and more than doubled in the Martian environment. This certainly suggests the presence of bacteria on Mars and perhaps on other celestial bodies—some of them possibly deadly to man.

Frequency and Area of Occurrence

Epidemics occur at erratic, unpredictable intervals. In the history of the human race up to 1920, disastrous epidemics probably have occurred at least once in each generation. Recently, there has been a marked reduction in frequency and severity, due primarily to the application of advanced techniques in public health, sanitation, and immunization. Epidemics occur all over the world. They are likely to be most severe where a relatively isolated population is suddenly exposed to a virulent microorganism.

Important Past Examples—U.S.A.

Date	Type	Place	Deaths*
1834	Cholera	New York City	827
1873	Cholera	U. S.	3,700
1919	Influenza	U. S.	550,000

Other Areas

Date	Type	Place	Deaths*
180 A.D.	Unknown	Rome	2,000 per day
500-550	Bubonic plague (Plague of Justinian)	Europe and Asia	100,000,000 (20-50%)
1098-1101	Unknown	Crusaders in Europe	280,000 (93%)
1348	Bubonic plague	World	25,000,000 (25-75%)
1349-1350	Bubonic plague	England	1,200,000 (20-30%)
1360-1361	Bubonic plague	Poland	(50%)
1418	Bubonic plague	Paris	50,000
1485	Sweating sickness	England	Thousands
1507	Sweating sickness	England	Thousands

* Showing in parentheses the estimated % of population killed.

Date	Type	Place	Deaths
1518	Sweating sickness	England	Millions (30-50%)
1520	Smallpox	Mexico	Several million (50%)
1529	Sweating sickness	England	Several million (30-50%)
1531	Measles	Mexico	Several hundred thousands
1545	Unknown	Mexico	1,000,000 (25-50%)
1551	Sweating sickness	England	not known
1603	Bubonic plague	London	34,000 (14%)
1628	Typhus	Lyons (France)	60,000
1628	Typhus	Limoges (France)	25,000
1663	Bubonic plague	Amsterdam	10,000 (5%)
1664	Bubonic plague	Amsterdam	24,000 (12%)
1665	Bubonic plague	London	69,000 (27%)
1675	Bubonic plague	Malta	11,000
1679	Bubonic plague	Vienna	76,000
1681	Bubonic plague	Prague	83,000
1711	Bubonic plague	Brandenburg	215,000
1711	Bubonic plague	Austria	300,000
1722	Bubonic plague	Marseilles	40,000 (33%)
1770	Bubonic plague	Moscow	80,000
1801-1803	Yellow fever	Haiti (French army)	22,000 (88%)
1831	Cholera	Moscow	4,500
1847	Typhus	Canada	20,000
1855-1856	Cholera	Crimea: French	49,000
		British	17,000
		Russian armies	37,000 (15%)
1867	Malaria	Mauritius	32,000
1875	Measles	Fiji Islands	40,000 (25%)
1894	Bubonic plague	Canton, China	100,000
1896-1936	Bubonic plague	India	12,000,000
1908	Malaria	India	1,000,000
1910	Bubonic plague	Manchuria	60,000
1910	Cholera	Russia	131,000
1915	Typhus	Serbia	150,000
1917-1923	Typhus	Russia	3,000,000 (2%)
1918-1919	Influenza	Worldwide	20,000,000
1919	Typhus	Poland	20,000
1920	Typhus	Poland	23,000
1920	Dysentery	Poland	5,000

Date	Type	Place	Deaths
1947	Cholera	Egypt	11,000
1964	Cholera	South Vietnam	300

Causes

The primary causes of epidemics are infectious microorganisms. Contributing causes have been poor health habits, bad sanitation, vectors, and overcrowding.

Possible Preventive Measures

An important preventive measure is vaccination—repeated at appropriate intervals. Also important are sound sanitary measures, and good health habits in the population. In the United States, the levels of general health and sanitation are quite high. However, our level of resistance to smallpox may be dangerously low. Almost all Americans have been vaccinated against smallpox at one time, but such vaccinations give adequate immunity for a limited time only. American troops in World War II and the Korean War died of smallpox, even though they had been vaccinated years before. If smallpox were brought into this country many Americans would contract it. The American Medical Association has recommended that all Americans maintain their levels of immunity to smallpox by periodic revaccination. Such revaccination should be at intervals of not more than five years ordinarily, and at intervals of one year if there has been exposure to smallpox.

Immunization against other diseases is also important. Routinely, most Americans are also immunized against diphtheria, tetanus, whooping cough, and poliomyelitis. Preventive immunizations against other diseases, such as typhoid fever, typhus, yellow fever, Rocky Mountain spotted fever, and cholera, are available for special risk groups, for travelers, and for everybody in the event of an epidemic.

Other preventive measures include purification of water, sanitary inspections of food-handling establishments, insect control, and proper sewage disposal systems. Case-finding and epidemiological tracing of contagious-disease spread are also of great importance.

At the individual level, sound basic health habits are important at all times but especially so during an epidemic. It should be emphasized that adequate rest and nutrition are vital hygienic measures and that they apply to doctors and nurses, too. During an epidemic, it would be a serious error for doctors and nurses to work overlong hours at the expense of proper rest. The end result would be detrimental, not only to themselves but to the community as a whole.

Another measure whose importance cannot be overestimated is to prevent the contamination of the earth by microorganisms from other celestial bodies. At the present, there seems to be no effective control of the activities of the National Aeronautic and Space Administration as regards the prevention of such contamination. Controls from within an organization of that sort are notoriously ineffective since they are subject to the policies of the group's leaders, who may be willing to accept risks that the general population would consider excessive. A single microscopic spore, brought back to earth inside a space vehicle, could wipe out all life on earth. The only effective preventive measure appears to be to abandon the plans to send people to the moon and to Mars, and instead plan to send unmanned instrumented vehicles which would radio data back to earth, but would not return themselves. This would have the added advantage of saving at least $10 billion.

Measures for Minimizing Casualties from Initial Impact

In some cases, it may be possible to immunize most of the remaining population in a large area after an epidemic has started. It would be helpful if we had stand-by facilities for making vaccines for new microorganisms which may produce epidemics.

We have antibiotics and chemotherapeutic agents for the bacteria and rickettsiae which cause epidemics, but not for the viruses. It is not clear whether the quantity of antibiotics stockpiled would be enough to handle a major epidemic.

There are also specific public health measures which would be helpful in minimizing most epidemics. They are too complex for coverage in this book, but the interested reader may consult one of the standard texts in public health.

Recognition and Warning Signs

Public health authorities are constantly on the alert for evidence of a beginning epidemic and will issue any necessary warnings.

Main Mechanisms of Death and Injury

These vary with the type of disease involved.

Prevention of Further Casualties after Initial Impact

The term "initial impact" here refers to the disease which started the epidemic. Past experience has shown that epidemics of one type of disease had so lowered the resistance of the general population that epidemics of other diseases, previously dormant or infrequent, developed and killed many more. Sometimes, the secondary epidemic killed more persons than the initial one. The prevention of a secondary epidemic may involve the entire catalogue of techniques of the public health departments and sanitarians. Included are immunization procedures, destruction of rats and insects, greater surveillance of food and water, and closer attention to sewage and garbage disposal. An important factor in preventing secondary epidemics of air-transmitted diseases is avoidance of overcrowding; adequate nutrition, clothing, shelter, and rest are also of life-saving importance.

Special Procedures and Problems in Rescue, First Aid, Evacuation, and Definitive Medical and Nursing Care

If an epidemic similar to those of the past should strike again, it might prove impossible to give the victims the type of care which seriously ill patients now receive in American and many other hospitals. It may be necessary to utilize the stockpiled civil defense hospitals and to utilize the services of partially trained volunteers. In the event of such occurrence, steps should be taken to prevent over-conscientious physicians, nurses, ancillary medical personnel and volunteers from overworking to an extent that lowers their own resistance and furnishes fertile soil for further epidemics.

chapter

32 EXPLOSIONS

General Description

An explosion is a sudden release of a large amount of energy, accompanied by shock and pressure waves. A very rapid burning can be an explosion. For example, if gasoline is mixed with air in the proper proportions and ignited, the burning is extremely rapid, and the expanding, heated products of combustion that move outward create damaging shock waves in the air. Other fuels, such as natural gas and coal dust, can also produce explosions when mixed with air.

Gunpowder is an example of materials that can explode by rapid burning without added air. Gunpowder contains its own oxygen in the form of nitrates and the carbon and sulfur combine with the oxygen in the nitrate, releasing large amounts of heat. When it is not enclosed, gunpowder tends to burn relatively slowly. However, if enclosed as in a cartridge, the beginning of the burning raises pressures and temperatures so high that the rest of the burning process takes place rapidly enough to constitute an explosion.

Another type of explosion is sometimes referred to as detonation. In a detonation, the material involved has the necessary gases already locked within its molecular structure. When set off by shock or heat, these molecules are suddenly rearranged to form masses of hot gas. This process takes place much more rapidly than the burning-type of explosion, so that the shock produced is much greater. Materials which can detonate include nitroglycerine, dynamite, ammonium nitrate, perchloric acid, picrates and picric acid, fulminate of mercury, and nitrocellulose.

We will not consider thermonuclear explosions in this chapter.

Frequency and Area of Occurrence

Fatal explosions have occurred all over the world, and their frequency is increasing because of the increased use of explosive materials in industry. It should be noted that these explosive materials are often employed for qualities other than their explosiveness. Perchloric acid, for instance, which detonated and killed 17 people in Los Angeles, was being used in an electroplating process.

The storage of potentially explosive gases under high pressure and low temperature can result in an explosion in the event a tank bursts, as it did in 1944 in Cleveland.

Important Past Examples—U.S.A.

Date	Place	Materials	Deaths
March 7, 1913	Baltimore, Maryland	Dynamite	55
September 27, 1915	Ardmore, Oklahoma	Gasoline	47
April 10, 1917	Eddystone, Pennsylvania	Munitions	133
July 2, 1918	Split Rock, New York	Munitions	50
May 22, 1919	Cedar Rapids, Iowa	Starch dust	44
March 18, 1937	New London, Texas (school)	Natural gas	294
Sept. 11, 12, 1940	Kenvil, New Jersey	Munitions	100
July 17, 1944	Port Chicago, California	Information not available	322
October 20, 1944	Cleveland, Ohio	Liquid gas	135
April 16, 1947	Texas City, Texas	Ammonium nitrate fertilizer	561
May 19, 1950	South Amboy, New Jersey	Ammunition	30
October 31, 1963	Indianapolis, Ind. (Coliseum)	Bottled gas	73

Other Areas

Date	Place	Materials	Deaths
December 6, 1917	Halifax, Canada	Munitions	1,600
August, 1947	Cadiz, Spain	Munitions	149
July 28, 1948	Ludwigshafen, Germany	Information not available	184
June, 1950	Syria	Gasoline	60
January, 1951	Peru	Dynamite	132
January, 1953	Valparaiso, Chile	Dynamite	57
August, 1953	Bengazi, Libya	Ammunition	50
August 7, 1956	Cali, Colombia	Dynamite	1,100
June, 1958	Santa Amaro, Brazil	Fireworks	110
March 4, 1960	Havana, Cuba	Munitions	100

In addition to these major disasters, there have been many smaller explosions in the United States and other nations, killing less than 25 persons each. The total deaths from all of these lesser explosions probably is much greater than the total from the larger explosions listed here.

Causes

Some explosions are caused by carelessness, others by inadequate knowledge of the explosive hazard of certain chemicals. The greatest explosion disaster in America, at Texas City, came about because apparently no one at the scene had realized that ammonium nitrate could detonate. The explosion at Halifax, Canada, was probably due to sabotage by German agents.

Possible Preventive Measures

Storage and use of potentially explosive materials should be restricted to areas well removed from residences, schools, and other areas where the general public is likely to be. When new chemicals are introduced, the burden of proof as to their safety should be on the user, instead of having fire department or law-enforcement agencies prove their explosiveness.

Stricter regulation of gasoline storage and transportation would probably be of value, since several fatal explosions have resulted from unsafe handling or transportation of large quantities of gasoline.

Measures for Minimizing Casualties from Initial Impact

The only practical measure for minimizing casualties is to keep people away from places where explosions may occur. Since several disastrous explosions, such as the one at Texas City, have followed fires, the public should be educated to stay away from fires and not to consider them as exciting, entertaining spectacles.

Recognition and Warning Signs

Except in the case of fires, there are no known signs of an impending explosion which would provide useful warning.

Main Mechanisms of Death and Injury

The major causes of death and injury are direct blast effects on the human body and the propulsion of debris at high velocities, causing penetrating and crushing effects. Burns also result from most explosions.

Prevention of Further Casualties after Initial Impact

An explosion may damage nearby containers of additional explosive material; this could lead to a series of additional explosions. An assessment of the situation, therefore, should be made by a trained explosive expert. If there is a real danger of additional explosions, rescue and first-aid workers should be kept out of the area until the firemen and explosive experts have control of the situation and indicate that it is safe to enter the area.

Special Procedures and Problems in Rescue, First Aid, Evacuation, and Definitive Medical and Nursing Care

A major rescue problem may be the difficulty in getting through piles of debris to find the victims. Many fractures and blast injuries will be encountered. Many of the surviving casualties will be deafened because of ruptured eardrums, so that communication with them may be difficult.

War time experience has helped solve many of the problems of definitive medical and nursing care of the injured.

33 FIRES—GENERAL

This chapter will consider the general features of all fires. In view of their importance, fires in schools, hospitals, and hotels will be discussed separately in the chapters that follow.

General Description

A fire is a chemical process in which fuel, raised to a kindling temperature, combines rapidly with oxygen or other supporters of combustion, evolving large amounts of heat. Three elements are needed for a fire—a combustible fuel, a supporter of combustion (usually oxygen) which combines with the fuel, and a high enough temperature to start the process. As long as all three elements are present, the fire will continue; if one is removed, it will cease. Most fires give off smoke which is highly toxic.

A *conflagration* is a fire which extends beyond its original area to engulf other areas. Usually, conflagrations are produced when wind conditions are favorable. Forest fires and fires involving several buildings are examples of conflagrations. Some conflagrations have involved areas of 1,800 *square miles.*

A *firestorm* is a fire in a large area which exhibits certain characteristics. The area of a firestorm usually measures more than 1 square mile. The many individual fires in the area coalesce into one huge flame, and the area becomes so hot that all combustibles begin to burn, even if no flame has reached them before. Temperatures of 1,000° to 2,000° F. are usual in the entire area outside of large buildings. The firestorm acts like a gigantic fireplace and chimney. The flames and hot gases move upwards, while surface winds blow in from all sides at velocities up to 50 miles per hour. As a result, firestorms seldom spread. On the other hand, once a firestorm starts there is no known way of stopping it. Toxic and lethal concentrations of carbon monoxide are present within the firestorm area; there is also a relative diminution of oxygen but this aspect has been grossly exaggerated. The oxygen levels in the firestorm area are sufficient for human needs (chapter 50). The killers are the heat and carbon monoxide levels, not the oxygen deprivation. Firestorms may be part of large conflagrations.

In general, a firestorm is hard to produce, even in warfare, and this would be true even with hydrogen bombs (chapter 50). To be involved in a firestorm, an area must be at least 20% under roof (or the equivalent in forest). Some experts believe that at least 30% must be under roof (chapter 50). Such conditions of extreme concentration of combustible building material are found only in a few areas of a few cities. Firestorm hazards have been greatly exaggerated in the lay press. In one of the worst firestorms known, that in Hamburg in World War II (chapter 50), fully 85% of the people in the firestorm area survived although some, in inadequate shelters, perished.

Fires are also classified in terms of the type of fuel involved.

A *class A* fire is one in which ordinary, solid combustible materials— like wood, paper, and rubber—are burning. These fires can be put out with water or any other type of extinguisher.

A *class B* fire is one in which liquids—such as oil, gasoline, and paint— are burning. Water, and soda acid extinguishers cannot be used effectively since they tend to spread the fire. There are some cases, however, in which professional firemen can use water to put out or contain such a fire.

A *class C* fire is one in which live electrical devices are involved. Water, soda acid and foam cannot be used because they cause short circuits and may make the fire worse.

As a fire spreads, however, it usually becomes a *class A* fire because of the solid fuel in the area.

There is still another type of fire which ought to be recognized and designated by a letter: let us call it *class X*. A *class X* fire would be one in which the oxygen or other supporter of combustion is already present in the fuel and need not be supplied from outside. Examples of such fuels would include nitrates, chlorates, and almost all explosive materials. The significance of such a classification is threefold. It would indicate, first, that since the oxygen is already present in the fuel mixture, the fire cannot be smothered by removing oxygen, and fire extinguishers and steam, therefore, become useless. (Sometimes, these fires can be put out by lowering the temperature with large volumes of cold water.) The second significance of such a classification would be the indication that such fires can suddenly become explosions. Thirdly, it would be a reminder that these fires often produce poisonous gases which are far more dangerous than the smoke from ordinary fires.

Class X fires are relatively unimportant when compared to class A, B, and C fires in terms of total number of fires. However, in terms of causing disasters, class X fires are important enough to warrant special attention. The Texas City explosion which killed over 500 people, started with a class X fire. The fire at the Crile Clinic, which killed over 100 people, probably started as a class X fire in nitrate-containing X-ray film. Modern industry today is using increasing amounts of materials which could support a class X fire.

There are serious misconceptions about some of the terms relating to fire resistance.

The term "fireproof" does not mean that a building is safe in case of fire, or that it cannot be involved in a fatal fire. A fireproof building is defined as a building whose structure will remain intact after a burn-out of its contents, i.e., its walls and roof will remain standing. A stove is an excellent example of a fireproof construction. A fireproof building can be a death-trap if it contains combustible materials, and if it has open stairwells and shafts. The Winecoff hotel in Atlanta was a fireproof building, yet over 100 people died in it. There have been several other examples of fatal fires in fireproof buildings.

The term "fire resistive" means that the structural members, holding the weight of the building (beams, etc.), will remain strong enough in a fire to prevent collapse for a substantial period of time. The danger to occupants, however, may be as great or greater than in a non-fire-resistive building.

Unfortunately, there are no terms in general use to denote whether or not a building is safe for its *occupants* in the event of fire.

Frequency and Area of Occurrence

Fires of various sizes occur daily in the United States. They kill an average of 10,000 persons a year, 2,000 of them children.* They occur in forests, farms, suburbs and cities, on ships, in shacks, and in fireproof buildings. Fires also follow other disasters, adding to the toll.

Important Past Examples—U.S.A.
(Excluding school, hospital and hotel fires)

Date	Place	Deaths
October 8, 1871	Chicago	250
October 9, 1871	Peshtigo, Wisconsin (forest)	1,152
December 5, 1876	Brooklyn, New York (theatre)	295
September, 1881	Minnesota (forest 1,800 *square miles*)	125+
September 1, 1894	Hinckley, Minnesota (forest)	413
June 30, 1900	Hoboken, New Jersey (dock)	326
September 20, 1902	Birmingham, Alabama (church)	115
December 30, 1903	Chicago (theatre)	602
June 15, 1904	U. S. ship, Gen. Slocum	1,030

* *Disaster, 1: 3, 1947.*

Date	*Place*	*Deaths*
January 4, 1908	Boyertown, Pennsylvania (theatre)	170
March 25, 1911	New York (Triangle factory)	145
October 12, 1918	Cloquet, Minnesota (forest, 2,000 *square miles*)	400-500
April 21, 1930	Columbus, Ohio (prison)	320
September 8, 1934	Steamship Morro Castle	125
April 23, 1940	Natchez, Mississippi (dance hall)	198
November 28, 1942	Boston (night club)	491
July 6, 1944	Hartford, Connecticut (circus)	168
December 19, 1960	Aircraft carrier Constellation	50

Other Areas

December 8, 1881	Vienna (theatre)	850
May 25, 1887	Paris (theatre)	200
September 4, 1887	Exeter, England (theatre)	200
May 4, 1897	Paris (bazaar)	150
June 20, 1919	Puerto Rico (theatre)	150
September 1, 1923	Tokyo and Yokohama (following earthquake)	100,000
January 21, 1934	Chinese ship	216
December 12, 1942	St. John's, Newfoundland (hostel)	99
August 30, 1947	Paris, France (theatre)	89
December 28, 1947	Hankow, China (riverfront)	500
September 23, 1948	Hong Kong (warehouse area)	135
September, 1949	Chungking, China	1,700
September 17, 1949	Noronic (Canadian ship in dock)	119
March 3, 1960	Pusan, Korea (chemical plant)	63
November 13, 1960	Syria (theatre)	152
March 15, 1961	Fukuoka, Japan (colliery)	26
December 17, 1961	Brazil (circus)	323

Causes

Most fires can be said to be caused by storing combustible material in such a way that it can be ignited. However, there are additional causal factors which determine whether a fire is readily extinguished, or whether it grows rapidly, killing many people. These additional causal factors (not necessarily in order of importance) include:

1. Poor building construction practices (often these are not visible after completion of the building and are rather technical, having to do with the layout of stairs, shafts, vents, and wires).

2. Political interference with preventive actions recommended by firemen.

3. Poor housekeeping in buildings—storage of inflammables without adequate precautions to prevent fires.

4. Inadequate or absent automatic sprinkler and warning systems.

5. Inadequate exits.

6. Overcrowding of buildings.

7. Delay in notifying the fire department.

8. Inadequate fire safety laws for buildings. A particular hazard comes from the absence of retroactive provisions, i.e., when stricter laws for fire safety are passed, no provisions are made for their application to buildings already erected. For this reason, older buildings are usually more hazardous.

9. Carelessness with matches, fires, cigarettes.

Possible Preventive Measures

1. Strict laws for proper fire-safe building construction.

2. Provisions to make fire safety laws retroactive for existing buildings —within reason—or to impose higher taxes on unsafe buildings. Such laws exist in Hartford, Connecticut.

3. Public support of fire departments whenever they ask for correction of hazardous conditions.

There are several examples where political interference with fire safety rules led to disaster. In a Massachusetts town, a fire inspector who reported many violations in a plant that made women's heels coated with nitrocellulose was immediately demoted since the mayor owned the plant. Six months later, an explosion in the plant killed 20 persons. Two months before the La Salle Hotel fire in Chicago, a fire inspector found ten violations. Some were removed but the major ones were still there when the fire broke out. In part, the death toll in the Hartford circus fire was due to political interference with efforts to have the canvas of the tent flame-proofed.*

4. Strict enforcement of maximum occupancy regulations.
5. Elimination of combustible decorations from interstate commerce.
6. Installation of automatic alarm and sprinkler systems.
7. Use of American rather than foreign ships for travel. Even older American ships are much safer in regard to fire than the more modern foreign luxury liners.

Measures for Minimizing Casualties from Initial Impact

Training everyone to be fire conscious.

Teaching people automatically to make note of exits as they enter a building.

Training in orderly evacuation of a building and avoidance of panic.

On-the-spot leadership to prevent panic when a fire starts in a crowded place.

Provision of adequate, modern equipment for all fire departments.

Recognition and Warning Signs

The sight or smell of smoke is the most important warning sign. Evacuation of the building should begin immediately and the fire department should be called. In some fires, escape routes were cut off within eight minutes of the first smell of smoke.

Main Mechanisms of Death and Injury

Most fire deaths are caused by inhalation of smoke and toxic gases, not by flames.

Prevention of Further Casualties after Initial Impact

It is important to prevent the spreading of a fire and a recurrence of it (flare-up).

Special Procedures and Problems in Rescue, First Aid, Evacuation, and Definitive Medical and Nursing Care

Rescue in a fire is ordinarily a job for trained firemen.

If the burned victim can be transported to a hospital within 30 minutes, first-aid measures may be omitted. If a delay of more than 30 minutes is anticipated, a "burn solution" may be made up and given to the patient to drink. This solution delays and may prevent the development of

* Kearney, P. W., *Disaster on Your Doorstep*. Harper and Bros., New York, 1953, pp. 14-18.

shock. It is made by adding 5.5 grams of table salt and 4 grams of bicarbonate of soda to a liter of water; lemon juice may be added for flavor. An adult patient should drink 400 cc. initially and 200 cc. every hour thereafter until hospitalized. A record of intake should be kept. Severe burn cases require more hours of surgeons' and nurses' time than any other injury or operation. They may also need specialized equipment such as an artificial kidney, which can only serve a few persons at a time. Therefore, most hospitals can handle only a relatively small number of severe burn cases efficiently. In one situation, 15 burn cases severely strained all the resources of a modern 800-bed hospital.

In other words, if there are a large number of burn cases in a small or moderate size town, immediate consideration should be given to distant evacuation of most of the victims. Burn cases can be moved by ambulance, train, or air during the first 24 hours. Afterwards, movement may be too hazardous. Therefore, if the number of burn cases seems beyond the capacity of the local hospitals (see chapter 16), it would be wise to plan on an evacuation to large cities such as St. Louis, New York, Chicago, and Los Angeles as soon as initial anti-shock therapy has been given.

34 FIRES—HOSPITALS AND NURSING HOMES

General Description

A hospital or nursing home fire poses special problems because many of the patients are helpless and unable to save themselves.

Frequency and Area of Occurrence

There were 80 fatal hospital fires between 1931 and 1953, or approximately four per year. The rate does not seem to have lessened. These fires have occurred in new as well as in old buildings. Non-fatal hospital fires occur at the rate of four per day.

Important Past Examples—U.S.A.

Date	Place	Deaths
May 15, 1929	Crile Hospital, Cleveland, Ohio	124
July 24, 1931	Home for Aged, Pittsburgh, Pennsylvania	48
April 5, 1949	St. Anthony's Hospital, Effingham, Illinois	77
January 7, 1950	Mercy Hospital, Davenport, Iowa	41
March 29, 1953	Nursing home, Largo, Florida	35
February 17, 1957	Home for Aged, Warrenton, Missouri	72
December 8, 1961	Hartford Hospital, Connecticut	16
November 23, 1963	Norwalk, Ohio	63

These do not include the many cases in which 15 or less people have died.

Other Areas: data is not available.

Causes

A basic cause of fatal hospital fires is poor construction. A fire expert estimates that 85% of the hospitals and sanitariums in the country are "built to burn."* So-called "fireproof" construction is not enough. Many of the hospital contents are inflammable, including mattresses, bedding, gases, and so forth. Because of the immobilized condition of many patients, ordinary emergency exits may not be sufficient.

Possible Preventive Measures

The most important single step in preventing fatal hospital fires would be the installation of automatic sprinkler-alarm systems.** These would probably prevent close to 98% of the fatalities that would otherwise occur. Such systems can be installed at a relatively low cost, and it is difficult to understand why so few hospitals have them.

Another important step would be the enclosure, and if necessary, the insulation of vertical passages, such as stairs, shafts, and laundry chutes so that fire in them cannot spread to other areas.

The use of any combustible material in hallways and corridors should be prohibited by law, and these laws should be made retroactive. The fire in the new, supposedly fireproof, Hartford Hospital in 1961 was fatal largely because a combustible acoustic ceiling caught fire. This type of ceiling has no place in a hospital—it is dangerous anywhere.

Regular, realistic fire drills for all personnel, including the night shifts, doctors and nurses, would also be of great benefit.

State laws should require monthly fire inspections by qualified fire inspectors who are not connected with the hospital, and whose reports will be made public within 48 hours.

Nurses, through their organizations, could have most of the hazardous fire conditions corrected. One way would be a listing by the nurses' organizations of the relative fire safety of each hospital and nursing home in their county, state, or region. Education of the public would be an additional method.

Measures for Minimizing Casualties from Initial Impact

Adequate fire escape facilities, suitable for bed-ridden patients, are difficult to add to some of the existing hospitals. However, in many cases it would be possible to give effective protection by installing fire doors so as to compartment each floor of the hospital. These fire doors should, ideally, be arranged in pairs, with a ten-foot space between them. Then, bed patients could be wheeled from the involved wing to a safe wing, without their passage creating a draft that might bring the fire along.

* Kearny, P. W. *Disaster on Your Doorstep.* Harper and Bros., New York, 1953, pp. 74-75.
** Guidelines to Hospital Fire Safety. *J. of Am. Hosp. Association,* Special Issue, Hospitals; June 1, 1962.

Training of all hospital personnel in fire-fighting, and the provision of adequate, periodically inspected fire extinguishing equipment would help to reduce fire fatalities and injuries.

Recognition and Warning Signs

The smell of smoke is an absolute indication for immediate notification of the hospital and city fire department. No one should ever have the authority to order or advise someone not to call the city fire department. Morally, no one should have the right to obey such an order if it were given.

A visitor at St. Anthony's Hospital in Effingham, Illinois, smelled smoke and reported it to the hospital authorities. However, it was not reported promptly to the city fire department. By the time the city firemen were notified and arrived, the fire was out of control.

Ideally, the hospital fire alarm system should be directly tied in to the city fire alarm, so that the city firemen are notified automatically. However, few hospitals seem to have such an arrangement.

Main Mechanisms of Death and Injury

Most deaths occur from inhalation of smoke and toxic vapors. Other deaths and injuries come from burns.

Prevention of Further Casualties after Initial Impact

Patients and hospital personnel trapped in a room during a hospital fire can often survive if they follow some basic procedures designed to keep smoke and flames out of their room. All doors, transoms, and vents should be kept closed. Wet cloths can be used to plug all cracks. Windows may be opened slightly from time to time to get some fresh air, provided this procedure does not draw smoke or hot air into the room.

Special Procedures and Problems in Rescue, First Aid, Evacuation, and Definitive Medical and Nursing Care

The rescue of bed-ridden patients from a burning hospital or nursing home is a major problem. However, some procedures have been worked out which may be useful.* They should be studied and rehearsed well in advance of the emergency. First aid, and definitive medical and nursing care problems are the same as in other fires (chapter 33).

* McGrath, R. *Emergency Removal of Patients and First Aid Fire Fighting in Hospitals.* National Safety Council and American Hospital Association. Chicago, 1956.

35   FIRES—HOTELS

General Description

Hotel fires cause deaths partially because of the large numbers of untrained persons who collect in an unfamiliar area.

Frequency and Area of Occurrence

Over a ten-year period it was found that hotels reported an average of four small fires each per year. There were probably others that went unreported. Most hotels are subject to fatal fires, including the so-called "fireproof" hotels. Indeed, the worst hotel fire in history took place in a "fireproof" hotel.

Important Past Examples—U.S.A.

Date	Place	Deaths
January 10, 1883	Newhall Hotel, Milwaukee, Wisconsin	71
March 17, 1899	Windsor Hotel, New York, New York	45
May 16, 1938	Terminal Hotel, Atlanta, Georgia	35
September 7, 1943	Gulf Hotel, Houston, Texas	55
June 5, 1946	LaSalle Hotel, Chicago, Illinois	61
December 7, 1946	Winecoff Hotel, Atlanta, Georgia	119
January 6, 1961	Thomas Hotel, San Francisco, California	20
November 18, 1963	Hotel, Atlantic City, New Jersey	25
December 29, 1963	Hotel, Jacksonville, Florida	22

Other Areas: information is not available.

Causes

   The actual initial cause of most fatal hotel fires appears to be carelessness—usually on the part of a guest. However, with sound fire-defense practices such fires would not be serious. The reasons that these fires become disasters include:

1. The use of inflammable hall carpets, drapes, wall coverings, and ceilings.
2. Open stair wells, elevator shafts, and ventilating ducts.
3. Lack of automatic sprinkler systems.
4. Delay in reporting the fire.

Possible Preventive Measures

The installation of automatic sprinkler systems is the major preventive measure. It could reduce fatalities by as much as 98%.

All open stairways, shafts, and ducts should be enclosed. In the Winecoff hotel fire the heat and flames raced up the open stairs. The fire started on the third floor. By the time firemen arrived a few minutes later, people were dying on floors up to and including the 15th floor.

There should be adequately protected exits which are never to be locked.

There should be adequate fire alarms throughout the hotel which guests can reach and ring.

All hotel employees should be trained in fire prevention and fire fighting.

Strict fire prevention laws for hotels should be passed and made applicable to buildings already constructed. This was done in Hartford, Connecticut, and is apparently quite legal and constitutional.

Measures for Minimizing Casualties from Initial Impact

The measures listed as preventive would also be of major value in minimizing casualties if prevention failed.

Recognition and Warning Signs

The smell of smoke in a hotel is an absolute indication for notification of the hotel management *and the city fire department*. A guest who smells smoke should telephone the city fire department personally, without delay; he should then help arouse and evacuate other guests. Do not rely on the hotel management to call the city fire department, and do not be deterred by being told the city fire department will be notified by the hotel management.

Main Mechanisms of Death and Injury

Most deaths are caused by inhalation of smoke and toxic vapors. Some deaths and injuries are due to burns, others to jumping out of windows. Some deaths occur when people, trying to slide down ropes or knotted sheets slide too fast, burn their hands by friction, and then let go.

Prevention of Further Casualties after Initial Impact

A guest, trapped in a hotel fire, can often survive by keeping calm and remembering some simple procedures.

If you suspect a fire is in progress, do not open your door until you check its temperature. Put your palm against the door at a level above your head. If the door feels hot, do not open it. The heat in the corridor probably is already too great for you to get to an exit alive. If the door seems warm, but not hot, open it just a crack, with your foot braced against it to keep it from suddenly flying open. Look through the crack. If you see heavy smoke, close the door quickly and also close the transom. Calk all cracks around the doors and transom with wet towels, etc., and keep them wet. Windows may be opened slightly for air. Wait for the firemen to rescue you.

Special Procedures and Problems in Rescue, First Aid, Evacuation, and Definitive Medical and Nursing Care

These are basically the same as in other fires (chapter 33).

36 FIRES—SCHOOLS

General Description

School fires include those occurring in public, private and parochial schools from the elementary to the university level.

Frequency and Area of Occurrence

There are approximately eight school fires per day in the United States. Fortunately, most have been easily extinguished and others have taken place at night so that we have been spared many tragedies. Each year, an average of 30 schools are totally destroyed by fire, showing that the relative infrequency of major loss of lives is a matter of luck rather than of safe school construction. Over the past half-century, average annual loss of life in school fires has amounted to 18 persons, including teachers and firemen.*

Private schools are considered particularly dangerous.

Important Past Examples—U.S.A.

Date	Place	Deaths
March 4, 1908	Collinwood, Ohio	176
May 18, 1923	Camden, South Carolina	77
December 24, 1924	Hobart, Oklahoma (one room)	36
March 19, 1937	New London, Texas (+ explosion)	294
December 1, 1958	Chicago, Illinois	95
March 5, 1959	Arkansas (near Little Rock)	24

Other Areas: no data available.

---

* Finchum, R. N. and Boerrigter, G. C. *School Fires: Prevention, Control, Protection.* U. S. Department of Health, Education, and Welfare, Washington, D. C., 1962, p. 10.

Causes

Disastrous school fires have been caused by one or more of the following:

1. Locked exits. The loss of 176 lives in the Lakewood School at Collinwood, Ohio, was the result of a locked exit door. Bodies were piled 12 feet high beyond the door. A clergyman, who was an eyewitness and who later left the ministry to do fire prevention work, reported 40 years later that ". . . we are still sending millions of our children to institutions that are no better than was that grammar school in Collinwood where 176 lives were snuffed out!"*

Despite this example, a competent fire inspector reported that relatively new schools have had padlocks on fire escape chutes, and faulty "panic bolts" on exit doors, so that able-bodied men couldn't open them.

2. Poorly planned design, with open stairways and vents and ducts. State laws vary greatly in their stringency.

3. Poor housekeeping, with inflammable materials kept inside the school.

4. Lack of interest in fire prevention. An investigator writing to the heads of state boards of education received an impudent letter from the head of the board in South Carolina, saying his board needed no advice from outsiders. A month later, a school fire killed 77 persons in that state.

Possible Preventive Measures

1. Better school design, with as much attention paid to safety as to architectural and teaching frills, would be helpful. At slight extra cost, schools can be made much safer not only against fires, but also against earthquakes and tornadoes.

2. Thorough periodic unannounced fire inspections of each school, public and private, should be conducted by experts from outside areas. To avoid political pressures, arrangements could be made whereby the fire chief of town A inspects schools of town B monthly, while the fire chief of town B inspects schools of town C, and so forth. This sort of arrangement should be set up by law on a state-wide basis.

3. Laws in each state are needed, making it a felony for anyone to lock any *exit* from a school while school is in session, unless tested, well-functioning "panic bolt" opening-arrangements are available.

4. Regulations should require each school principal to check each exit from his school every day to make sure that it opens readily.

* Kearney, P. W. *Disaster on Your Doorstep.* Harper and Bros., New York, 1953, p. 107.

Measures for Minimizing Casualties from Initial Impact

Well-planned and conducted fire drills are of major importance. A special type of fire drill, used in Texas and called the "blocked" fire drill, would be of even more value than ordinary drills. In a blocked fire drill, one exit is symbolically blocked by a red ball and no one is allowed to use it. No hint is given beforehand as to which exit is to be blocked. The teachers and students must then go out a secondary exit. This provides invaluable training in the use of a secondary exit when the primary one is cut off. After the Texas City explosion of 1947, the Danforth elementary school, over two miles away, was badly damaged, and almost every child was cut by flying glass. The bottom of one stairway was blocked by rubble. Nevertheless, the second-floor pupils were able to follow hand signals, turn back from the blocked exit, and go out through another exit at the other end of the building without panic and in an orderly fashion.

The value of blocked fire drills seems so clear that it is difficult to see why other states do not require them. Perhaps parents, through the PTA's, should take the initiative in having blocked fire drills in their own schools. It would be advisable for a committee of parents to time the drills. If a school cannot be completely evacuated in a short time with any one exit blocked, it is unsafe and should be abandoned.

Every older child, and every adult working in a school should be taught how to turn in an alarm. Furthermore, it should be emphasized that a false alarm, turned in *in good faith* is not to be criticized. This precaution is needed because some persons, afraid of turning in a false alarm, might delay too long after smelling or seeing smoke.

Recognition and Warning Signs

The smell of smoke is an absolute indication for an immediate sounding of the fire alarm and for evacuation of the school building, without taking any time out for consultation. In the Chicago school fire of 1958, the smell of smoke was detected at 2:30 P.M. Between 2:30 and 2:31 P.M., the teachers conferred; between 2:32 and 2:33 a teacher ran to the office. No one was there. Evacuation did not start until 2:35. The school building fire alarm was not pulled until 2:38, and the fire department was not notified until 2:41. When the firemen arrived at 2:44, the corridors were already unusable and the pupils were jumping out of windows. The delay of eight minutes in pulling the school fire alarm was probably fatal. Had the alarm been pulled at 2:31, the chances are that all would have survived.

Main Mechanisms of Death and Injury

The major cause of death is usually inhalation of smoke and toxic vapors. Burns also are a cause of death and injury. Some injuries are caused by jumping from windows.

Prevention of Further Casualties after Initial Impact

This is not likely to prove a problem in school fires.

Special Procedures and Problems in Rescue, First Aid, Evacuation, and Definitive Medical and Nursing Care

These are, in general, similar to those for most fires (chapter 33).

chapter

37   FLOODS

General Description

A flood is an overflowing of water beyond its usual confines in lakes, rivers, or oceans. Floods along seacoast areas are generally caused by different processes than floods in inland areas.

Frequency and Area of Occurrence

Floods of disaster magnitude on seacoast areas in the United States generally are associated with hurricanes, which are discussed in chapter 39 Sometimes a tsunami (discussed in chapter 46) causes flooding of a coastal area. In Holland, coastal floods have resulted from unusually high tides, and from breaks in dikes.

Inland floods of moderate magnitude occur almost every year in the United States and at least as often elsewhere in the world. At irregular intervals, averaging once every 50 years, flooding of much greater intensity than usual is likely to occur almost anywhere, including the United States.

Important Past Examples—U.S.A.

Date	Place	Deaths
May 3, 1889	Johnstown, Pennsylvania (dam collapse)	2,200
March 25-27, 1913	Ohio and Indiana	732
March 13, 1928	Santa Paula, California (dam collapse)	450
January 22 and 23, 1937	Ohio and Mississippi Valleys	250

In addition, most of the deaths in hurricanes have resulted from the accompanying floods.

Other Areas, principally after World War II

1887	China	900,000
1911	China	100,000
July, 1947	China	1,000
August, 1947	Honshu, Japan	2,000
September, 1947	India	1,000
May, 1948	China	330

152

Date	Place	Deaths
June, 1948	Turkey	90
June, 1948	China	3,500
September, 1948	Japan	858
December, 1948	Brazil	600
May, 1949	Brazil	200
June, 1949	Mexico	54
July, 1949	China	57,000
October, 1949	Guatemala	500
September, 1950	India	270
January, 1951	Morocco	70
May, 1951	Formosa	300
July, 1951	Japan	250
August, 1951	Manchuria	4,800
November, 1951	Iran	225
November, 1951	Italy	150
July, 1952	Japan	50
September, 1952	Philippines	74
January 31, and February 1, 1953	Holland and Western Europe	2,000
February, 1953	Indonesia	82
June, 1953	Japan	1,000
August, 1953	Iran	265
October, 1953	Spain	50
July, 1954	Tibet	300
August, 1954	Iran	150
August, 1954	Pakistan	300
August, 1954	Nepal	1,000
August, 1954	Iran	2,000
October, 1954	Italy	320
October, 1955	India and Pakistan	1,700
December, 1955	India	120
May, 1956	Haiti	50
July 24, 1956	Iran	300
July, 1956	Iran	900
August, 1956	Pakistan	200
August, 1956	Turkey	140
July, 1957	Philippines	1,000
July, 1957	China	550
July, 1957	Kyushu, Japan	513
July, August, 1957	South Korea	208
September, 1957	Pakistan	75
September, 1957	Turkey	90
September, 1957	Iran	120

Date	*Place*	*Deaths*
September, 1957	India	90
October, 1957	Spain	100
November, 1957	India	50
December, 1957	Ceylon	300
July, 1958	Argentina	350
April, 1959	Madagascar	143
May, 1959	South Africa	60
June, 1959	China	187
June, 1959	Colombia	184
July, 1959	Pakistan	100
July, 1959	South Korea	62
July, 1959	India	139
August, 1959	Taiwan	1,000
September, 1959	India	500
November, 1959	Mexico	2,000
December, 1959	France	323
September, 1959	Brazil	100
March, 1960	Brazil	100
September, 1960	India	256
September, 1960	Italy	36
October, 1960	Nicaragua	325
July, 1961	India	227
October, 1961	India	1,000
November, 1961	Somaliland, Africa	100
February, 1962	Germany	309
August, 1962	Colombia	134
August, 1962	India	27
September, 1962	South Korea	290
September, 1962	India	73
September, 1962	Spain	800
April, 1963	Afghanistan	107

Causes

The causes of most seacoast floods are discussed in the chapters on hurricanes and tsunamis. Inland floods are caused by other factors. Several disastrous floods have resulted from a sudden break in a dam which released enormous amounts of water on areas below the dam.

Usually, floods are caused by heavy rains or thaws of accumulated snows, or both. These factors may be aggravated by poor land conservation practices. If land is improperly plowed and farmed, it will not hold as much moisture as if it were properly managed land, and floods are likely to be more frequent and more severe. On the other hand, the really great floods which occur at relatively rare intervals are not preventable by land management practices, since they involve amounts of water which are much greater than the amounts the best-managed soil can accommodate.*

Possible Preventive Measures

Inland floods can be partially prevented or at least made less severe by good soil management practices. In certain areas, the building of dams may help prevent flooding. On the other hand, since a broken dam can result in a greater loss of life than most floods, dams should be designed with enough strength to make breakage impossible.

Measures for Minimizing Casualties from Initial Impact

Training and education of the population to obey flood warnings are essential.

It is also important to avoid the building of homes and businesses on the flood plains of rivers—the so-called "bottom land." These lands with their fertile soils may be used for farming, but the farm house itself should be situated on higher land. At irregular intervals, these flood plains, which may be several miles in width, will be covered by flood waters. We may say that in a period of 5,000 years approximately 100 great floods will cover the entire flood plain to a depth of many feet. However, we cannot predict the time when these floods will occur; two may take place only a year apart, and then the next one may not occur for another 100 years.

Recognition and Warning Signs

Floods resulting from heavy rains can usually be predicted by most of the area's residents. The problem here is not the lack of warning, but the tendency of some people to ignore the warning because they have experienced other, smaller floods in the past.

* Leopold, L. B. and Langbein, W. B. *A Primer on Water.* Superintendent of Documents, U. S. Government Printing Office, Washington, D. C., 1960, p. 29.

Main Mechanisms of Death and Injury

Drowning causes many deaths from floods. Some injuries and deaths are caused by direct trauma from floating debris carried along by the swift current.

Surprisingly, there may in some cases be a substantial number of casualties due to fire. A survivor of the Johnstown flood—a man who later became a well-known physician—reported that he saw many people burn to death in the ruins of buildings. Apparently, the wall of water which smashed Johnstown passed through in a relatively short time and did not thoroughly soak the timbers of those buildings. At the same time, burning coal in stoves and ovens was not completely extinguished by the flood and ignited the wood, starting conflagrations which killed many who were trapped in the debris.

Floods also may break large oil and gasoline storage tanks, and the film of oil and gasoline on the water may become ignited from one cause or another, spreading fire through a large area. In the flood which struck Kansas City, Missouri, in July, 1951, several large gasoline storage tanks were knocked loose and floated down the river. Escaping fuel caught fire, and for a time it looked as if a major part of Kansas City would be destroyed. Only the heroic efforts of the Kansas City firemen kept the incident from becoming a major disaster.

In addition, since floods contaminate water supplies, epidemics may become a major problem.

Prevention of Further Casualties after Initial Impact

An important preventive measure would be a set of laws, prohibiting installation of gasoline and oil storage tanks on flood plains of rivers, or other areas which could be affected by flooding.

Since the danger of having such storage facilities in a vulnerable area is clearly evident, the owners of facilities which have already been installed on flood plains should be held financially liable for any damage caused by the breaking loose or leakage of their tanks during a flood. The resulting increase in their insurance premiums would make a move to a safer location seem economically attractive.

Since floods, by contaminating water sources, make epidemics more likely, strict public health preventive measures are vital. We have been able to avoid secondary epidemics after recent American floods largely because of vigorous and effective action by public health authorities. Similar vigilance and effectiveness are essential in all future disasters.

Special Procedures and Problems in Rescue, First Aid, Evacuation, and Definitive Medical and Nursing Care

A major problem is rescue of the stranded inhabitants of the area, as well as of trapped motorists. The most practical solution to this problem appears to be the use of special amphibious vehicles and helicopters. The latter, of course, will have to be provided by the armed forces. It may prove practical to assign amphibious vehicles permanently to specially trained civil defense units near major rivers.

General Description

Highway accidents involve collisions between two or more moving vehicles or between a moving vehicle and a stationary object. Most individual highway accidents cause the deaths of a few people at a time. However, the yearly total of highway accident deaths and injuries is so high that the overall situation may properly be considered a major disaster, with the toll distributed over the entire year. On this basis, the approach to the highway accident problem is similar to the approach to other disasters.

Frequency and Area of Occurrence

The frequency of highway accidents is so high as to be an almost continuous process: before the victims of one crash can be transported to the hospital, several other crashes have taken place somewhere else in the nation. The yearly death toll is about 40,000 and the serious injuries come to more than a quarter of a million. Put into other terms, the *daily* death rate from these accidents is over 100, or about one death every 15 minutes. Thus, highway accidents constitute a major disaster every day.

Most highway deaths occur in the United States, largely because of our large volume of automobile traffic.

Important Past Examples: none.

Causes

There are several causes of highway accidents. The relative importance of each cause is not clear, and this entire field requires much more extensive research.

One cause is the design of roads. Many roads are too narrow, too winding, or too hilly for the high-speed traffic which uses them. The forward visibility of the drivers is inadequate because of the curves and hills. Even a careful driver may be killed if he rounds a curve or comes over a brow of a hill at a legal speed and finds a stopped vehicle in his path.

The design of motor vehicles is also a factor in causing accidents. Modern vehicles are so low that the driver's head is usually below the point it would reach if he were walking; this makes it difficult to see over minor hills on the road, and seriously reduces his forward vision. Also, since the vehicle itself is so low, it is difficult for other drivers to see it on a hilly road. The accent on comfort and style may also contribute to accidents, since a good deal of the "road feel" is sacrificed to fancy design.

The advertising of automobiles probably plays an important role in the high accident rate. Directly and subtly, the major automobile manufacturers imply that their cars are built for racing. Their television commercials feature the speed and power of their vehicles. The names chosen for the models often suggest speed (i.e., Thunderbird, Impala, Comet, Dart). They advertise enormous horsepower.

Other advertising campaigns are designed to appeal to a purchaser's latent hostilities. The automobile is presented in terms of power and weaponry. The psychological implication is that the owner will derive power over others in some mystical fashion. One company, in large billboard ads, compared its vehicle to a tiger. Another uses the name "Le Sabre" for one of its models, and "Cutlass" and "Wildcat" for others. Unfortunately, the subconscious mind is a dangerous object to try to manipulate for commercial purposes. It can, at the wrong second, be stimulated to a reaction which leads to an accident. Consider, for example, a man whose daily frustrations have led to a certain level of suppressed hostility. He purchases a car, selecting a vehicle which has subtly been presented to him as an instrument of power and force. As he drives along, he may suddenly find himself in a tight situation and act out his latent hostility by refusing to yield the right of way, thus causing an accident. There is growing evidence that many accidents result from inner hostility of one or the other driver, which for a split second is uncontrolled. It is not unreasonable to deduce that advertising campaigns which cater to people's hostility feelings by presenting cars as weapons, contribute to accidents.

Alcohol is another important factor in automobile accidents. In many of the accidents in which alcohol is involved, the driver was not drunk. He only had one or two drinks. However, even a small amount of alcohol tends to influence judgment, making accidents more likely.

To some extent, the use of vehicles in unsatisfactory operating condition also contributes to accidents. Bad brakes and worn tires probably cause a substantial number of deaths. Some used-car dealers are in the habit of taking tires which are worn smooth and cutting new grooves into them so that they look new—a particularly dangerous practice since these tires are much more likely to develop blow-outs than new tires or recaps.

The role of speed in causing accidents is not clear. Certainly, many accidents result from traveling too fast for road conditions. However, it has been reported that many fatal crashes take place at speeds between 30 and 40 miles per hour. Unfortunately, the reports do not specify how the speed was measured nor whether it was measured when the accident started, or when the impact occurred. For example, let us assume that a driver going 60 miles per hour suddenly sees a stalled truck ahead of him, applies his brakes, and slows to 30 miles per hour when his car hits the truck and he is killed. Is that considered a death resulting from a speed of 60 miles per hour or 30? In the absence of this sort of knowledge, it is not possible to determine the exact importance of speed in causing accidents.

Distraction of drivers by billboard advertising may contribute to some accidents, although there is no real evidence to prove this.

Possible Preventive Measures

Improvement in roads, increased visibility, and making passing safer should help to reduce accidents.

Safer car design, featuring increased height and better "road feel" would also be helpful.

Government regulation—either state or federal or both—of some of the automobile industry practices seems necessary. Some action is needed to stop the horsepower race, and the attempts to sell cars by presenting them as racers or as instruments of force and power. One is naturally reluctant to advocate any increase in government regulations. However, in view of the magnitude of the daily disasters, such a recommendation must reluctantly be made. After all, there are strict laws relating to the sale and possession of submachine guns. Yet the fact is that automobiles are far more deadly than submachine guns. Actually, more Americans have been killed by automobiles than by all the machine guns, cannons, rifles, bombs, torpedoes, and other weapons of our enemies in all the wars of our history.

Stricter regulation of billboards might also be of some value.

State laws prohibiting the cutting of new grooves in worn tires would prevent some accidents. Wisconsin has recently passed such a law.

There is no evidence whatever that the periodic warnings and exhortations to drive more carefully have any effect.

A major problem in the search for methods to reduce the extent of highway disasters is the scarcity of reliable information. This area merits a much greater research effort than is now in progress. Furthermore, the research should be sponsored and paid for by some government agency—not by the automobile companies—so that the results would be objective and the recommendations carry more weight.

There is one unusual feature in the reporting of highway accidents, and this may well represent one important gap in our knowledge. Most newspapers, in reporting automobile accidents, do not give the make of the car involved. The stories carry the names and addresses of the victims, the witnesses, and sometimes even of the investigating policeman. They may say that the car was a sedan, coupe, convertible, or station wagon, but they don't disclose its make. This is a curious omission, since in stories about firearms tradenames are often mentioned; newspapers frequently indicate that a Colt, a Winchester, a Remington, or any other make of gun was involved. Similarly, in airplane crashes, the make of the plane is reported.

This gap in reporting has been noted in most of the large newspapers. A few of the smaller papers do, however, give a complete story.

Measures for Minimizing Casualties from Initial Impact

The major measure is the installation and *use* of seat belts. Well-conducted tests have shown that seat belts could save many lives. Further research is needed on ways of improving seat belts.

A second important measure is the design of the car interior so that an occupant cannot be flung against a protuberance or a sharp edge. The best type of padding is one which will absorb the shock, as, for instance, certain foam plastics do. Rubber, which absorbs and then returns the force of a blow, is much less satisfactory.

Improvement of the front-end of the car with some shock-absorbent construction features would probably reduce the injury to the occupants to a considerable extent and might cut the death toll by 50% or more.

It has been stated in the Journal of the American Medical Association that "a motor car can be easily designed and built to prevent death and injury in all but the most severe crashes."* It has also been pointed out that the stopping distance of a car is a most important factor in the death rate. The stopping distance is the distance which the main part of the car travels after its front-bumper strikes a solid barrier, like a concrete abutment. It is usually equivalent to the distance between front-bumper and front-end of the engine block, or about one foot. If this distance were increased to two feet, it would save many lives now lost in accidents. Unfortunately, the advice of the medical profession often goes

* Campbell, H. E. Seat Belts. *J. A. M. A.*, March 11, 1961, p. 934.

unheeded by the automobile manufacturers until many years have gone by. Usually, it has taken some action by state legislatures to force manufacturers to pay more attention to safety features.

There is another aspect of the automobile industry's advertising policies that may be worth mentioning. It is common for manufacturers to point to the performance of their stock cars in special races, even though these cars are not really the same type as those purchased by the public. Stock cars used for racing have special safety equipment added, including heavy duty brakes, which are not part of the regular equipment of a car sold to the public. To enlighten the public about these differences may be one of a number of constructive steps that need to be taken in this area.

Recognition and Warning Signs

Any malfunction of an automobile should be considered a warning of a potential accident and should be corrected at once.

There are no other effective warning signs of an impending accident which can be relied upon.

Main Mechanisms of Death and Injury

Most deaths and injuries come from the sudden decelleration after the crash, when the head and body of the victim are slammed against a hard part of the car, such as the windshield or dashboard. A few deaths come from crushing injuries. Only a fraction of 1% of the deaths and injuries result from fires or entrapment, so that there need be no reluctance to use seat belts for fear that it might take an extra two seconds to get out of the vehicle.

Prevention of Further Casualties after Initial Impact

Warning signs should be put up at once for some distance on both sides of the crash area. This will help prevent additional vehicles from crashing into the original wrecks.

Special Procedures and Problems in Rescue, First Aid, Evacuation, and Definitive Medical and Nursing Care

Casualties from automobile accidents are so common that all police departments and general hospitals have considerable experience in dealing with them.

39 HURRICANES

General Description

A hurricane is a rotary storm, involving a wide area with winds exceeding 73 miles per hour. The winds rotate counter-clockwise in the northern hemisphere, and clockwise in the southern hemisphere. Hurricanes develop over ocean areas, causing maximum destruction when they hit seacoast areas. In the western Pacific area, the term used for this type of storm is "typhoon." Hurricanes originating in the Atlantic ocean usually move in a westerly or northwesterly direction until they approach the continent, when they tend to move more northerly. However, the exact path of a hurricane is not completely predictable, and hurricanes have doubled back and crossed their own track.

The usual forward speed of a hurricane circle is 10 to 15 miles per hour at first, but subsequently may increase to 25 miles per hour or more. The circular winds spin at over 73 miles per hour, regardless of the forward velocity of the entire circle.

Like all circular storms, a hurricane, in passing a particular point, seems to have three phases. First, there are high winds in one direction. Next, there is a clear phase, called the "eye". The eye of a hurricane is several miles wide—up to 50 in diameter—and quite calm. (By contrast, the center of a tornado is much smaller, and therefore exerts suction). Finally, there is the third phase with high winds blowing in a direction opposite to the initial one.

A hurricane has a track several thousand miles long, and several hundred miles wide. It can involve the entire Atlantic coast of the United States. It may persist five days along the coast.

The forces involved in a hurricane are enormous by any standard. A single hurricane releases forces much greater than could be released by all the hydrogen bombs in the world.

Frequency and Area of Occurrence

Several hurricanes a year develop over the Atlantic; they are generally identified by girls' names. In any particular year, only one or two are likely to strike the American coast full-force. Really disastrous hurricanes strike the United States less often than once a year. The vulnerable areas

are those near the seacoast, particularly if the elevation is only a few
feet above sea level.

Important Past Examples—U.S.A., after World War I

Date	Place	Deaths
September 18, 1926	Gulf coast of U. S.	372
September 12-17, 1928	Florida (and West Indies)	4,000
September 21, 1938	New England	600
August 30, 1954	Northeastern U. S.	68
September 11, 1954	Northeastern U. S. and Canada	23
October 12-16, 1954	Eastern U. S. and Haiti	347
August 12-13, 1955	Mid-southern coastal states	43
August 18-19, 1955	Eastern U. S.	400
June 27-30, 1957	Louisiana and Texas	430
September 4-12, 1960	Eastern U. S. and Caribbean	148
September 11, 1961	Louisiana and Texas	40

Other Areas: records are incomplete.

October 7, 1737	Bengal, India	300,000
October 20, 1926	Cuba	600
September 3, 1930	San Domingo	2,000
October 15-16, 1942	Bengal, India	11,000
November, 1946	Philippines	500
October, 1947	Hong Kong	1,000
February, 1948	Reunion Island	300
June, 1948	China	200
September, 1948	Japan	541
June, 1949	Japan	106
August, 1949	China	1,000
September, 1950	Japan	250
August, 1951	Jamaica	154
October, 1951	Japan	448
October 21, 1952	Philippines	440
September 25-27, 1953	Viet Nam and Japan	1,300
August, 1956	China	2,000
September 27-28, 1958	Japan	615

Date	*Place*	*Deaths*
August 20, 1959	China	720
September 17-19, 1959	Japan and Korea	2,000
September 26-27, 1959	Japan	4,500
October 27, 1959	Mexico	2,000
June 27, 1960	Philippines	100
July 31, 1960	Formosa	100
May 5, 1961	East Pakistan	185
September 12, 1961	Formosa	100
September 17, 1961	Japan	110
October 21, 1961	British Honduras	400
September 1, 1962	Hong Kong	64
October 6, 1963	Haiti	4,000

Causes

The causes of hurricanes are not known.

Possible Preventive Measures

Although experiments are in progress, there is as yet no known way to prevent the development of a hurricane.

Measures for Minimizing Casualties from Initial Impact

Early warnings of a probable hurricane, together with early, orderly, efficient evacuation of population from low-lying coastal areas to inland areas of greater elevation have already saved hundreds of lives.

Better training of the public in the importance of early evacuation is still needed.

Recognition and Warning Signs

Recognition activities are carried on by the U. S. Navy, the Coast Guard, and the Weather Bureau. They can recognize a hurricane days before it strikes the coast, and track it. The weather bureau gives timely and adequate warning over the radio. The efficiency of the warning system is such that virtually 100% of hurricane deaths are now preventable in the U. S.

Main Mechanisms of Death and Injury

Hurricane winds drive a wall of water before them. This raises the water level to as much as 16 or 18 feet above high tide. In low-lying coastal areas, a rapid general rise in sea level of this magnitude accompanied by even greater waves will cause drowning many miles inland of the usual coast. Most deaths in hurricanes have been drownings. Some deaths and injuries result from the caving-in of houses. When a hurricane strikes a swamp area, an additional danger may be presented by poisonous snakes which also seek protection, and may bite people in their path.

Prevention of Further Casualties after Initial Impact

People evacuated from danger areas should not be allowed to return until a competent official announces that the danger is over.

There may have been extensive damage to sanitary facilities, so that rigid measures will probably be needed to prevent epidemics. These measures may include purification of water and construction of emergency toilet facilities.

Special Procedures and Problems in Rescue, First Aid, Evacuation, and Definitive Medical and Nursing Care

The major rescue problem is that of locating and bringing to high land persons marooned by the rising waters. For this, special boats and amphibious vehicles with trained crews are often necessary.

The evacuation problem may be complicated by flooding of low sections of highways.

40 MINE DISASTERS

General Description

A mine disaster is a disaster which takes place in an excavation beneath the earth's surface. There are several types of mine disasters. In a cave-in, parts of the overlying rock fall down, blocking exits. In another type of situation known as "bumping," an overhanging roof breaks, and strata over the coal snaps back. This can also close exits. Many mine disasters are caused by explosions in the mine, either of coal dust or of methane gas.

Frequency and Area of Occurrence

The frequency of major mine disasters seems to be decreasing. To some extent, this results from safety measures, but it probably also reflects the fact that modern mining machinery makes it possible to operate with much fewer men. Thus, when a cave-in or explosion occurs, the number of dead now is much smaller. The average number of miners killed *per year* in accidents in coal mines alone, over a thirty-year period between 1911 and 1940, was about 1,900.

Important Past Examples—U.S.A., after 1900

Date	Place	Deaths
May 1, 1900	Scofield, Utah	200
May 19, 1902	Coal Creek, Tennessee	184
July 10, 1902	Johnstown, Pennsylvania	112
June 30, 1903	Hanna, Wyoming	169
January 25, 1905	Cheswick, Pennsylvania	179
February 20, 1905	Virginia City, Alabama	112
December 6, 1907	Monongah, West Virginia	361
December 19, 1907	Jacobs Creek, Pennsylvania	239
November 28, 1908	Marianna, Pennsylvania	154
November 13, 1909	Cherry, Illinois	259
April 8, 1911	Littleton, Alabama	128
October 22, 1913	Dawson, New Mexico	263
April 28, 1914	Eccles, West Virginia	181
October 27, 1914	Royaltown, Illinois	61
March 2, 1915	Layland, West Virginia	112
April 27, 1917	Hastings, Colorado	121

Date	Place	Deaths
February 8, 1923	Dawson, New Mexico	120
March 8, 1924	Castic Gate, Utah	171
April 28, 1924	Benwood, West Virginia	119
May 19, 1928	Mather, Pennsylvania	195
January 10, 1940	Bartley, West Virginia	92
March 25, 1947	Centralia, Illinois	111
December 21, 1951	West Frankfort, Illinois	119
February 4, 1957	Bishop, Virginia	37
December 6, 1962	Carmichaels, Pennsylvania	37
April 26, 1963	Clarksburg, West Virginia	22

Other Areas, primarily after World War II

Records are incomplete.

Information is sketchy but indicates that mine disasters are relatively more frequent, and kill more people, in areas other than the United States.

Date	Place	Deaths
December, 1914	Hokkaido, Japan	437
April, 1915	Shimonoseki, Japan	236
November, 1947	Saxony, Germany	96
October, 1949	Oberschlema, Germany	100
November, 1949	Zivickan, Germany	70
November, 1949	Johanngeorgenstadt, Germany	3,000
May, 1950	Gelsenkirchen, Germany	75
July, 1961	Prague, Czechoslovakia	180
November 9, 1963	Japan	over 500

Causes

Most mining disasters are caused by poor mining practices or by carelessness. In mining a shaft, vertical pillars are usually left to support the ceiling. If these pillars are inadequate, a cave-in may take place. Inadequate ventilation may result in explosive concentrations of coal dust or methane.

Possible Preventive Measures

These are often technical measures, in the domain of mining engineers and safety inspectors. As far as the general public is concerned, the principle preventive measures are the institution of strict safety rules for mining, and frequent inspection and enforcement by qualified personnel who have the complete support of all their superiors. At least one recent mine disaster occurred after a series of warnings about dangerous conditions and practices by a conscientious inspector were ignored by the mine owners, and by his own superiors.

Measures for Minimizing Casualties from Initial Impact

This is an area in which some research is needed. Many deaths have been due to asphyxiation. Some way of countering the toxic gases would be helpful.

Main Mechanisms of Death and Injury

These are asphyxiation and crushing.

Prevention of Further Casualties after Initial Impact

This has not been a problem in past mine disasters.

Special Procedures and Problems in Rescue, First Aid, Evacuation, and Definitive Medical and Nursing Care

Mine rescue is a highly technical procedure which should only be attempted by those with special training and equipment. There are seldom any special medical or nursing problems, since usually the victims are either dead or in relatively good condition. The ratio of injured to dead is quite low.

chapter

41 NUCLEAR REACTOR ACCIDENTS

General Description

A nuclear reactor accident is an occurrence in which an unplanned excess of heat or radiation in damaging quantities is released. The nuclear reactor accidents which have taken place thus far have been relatively minor in nature, involving only a few deaths and injuries. However, because of the potentiality of a major disaster, this type of accident deserves consideration. The Surgeon General of the United States has stated: "An accident in some types of industrial installations today, or in a nuclear reactor in the future, might pose a similar public health problem on the scale of a major disaster."*

Frequency and Area of Occurrence

The exact frequency of nuclear accidents is not known because, in all nations, government agencies responsible for nuclear reactor programs tend to be somewhat secretive as regards this topic. The areas involved in future nuclear accidents would be areas in the vicinity of reactors, and areas in which radioactive materials, including wastes, are stored.

Important Past Examples—U.S.A.

Date	Place	Deaths
January 3, 1961	Arco, Idaho	3

Other Areas

October 10, 1957	Windscale, Great Britain	1
Unknown	Mexico City	4

* Burney, L. E. Public Health Problems in Major Disasters. *Ann. Am. Acad. Pol. and Soc. Sci., 309:* 80, 1957, p. 80.

Causes

The possible causes of a nuclear reactor accident include errors in design or construction, human errors in handling the reactor, inadequate consideration of the effects of aging on the reactor and its components, and deliberate sabotage. Contributory causes may be the over-optimistic statements and press releases of AEC officials on the safety of their operations.

Another type of related accident would result from leakage of radioactive wastes from sealed, buried containers. Our information on this is scanty, but it seems that the problem is a serious one, since some of these wastes remain highly radioactive for hundreds of years, and are now accumulating in great quantities.

Possible Preventive Measures

One of the most important preventive measures would be the development by the appropriate agencies of a policy of complete honesty and objectivity in regard to the risks inherent in their projects and programs. It would then be possible to plan proper preventive measures in a realistic fashion. Unfortunately, in the past, announcements about the safety of certain nuclear programs have turned out to be erroneous and misleading.

A second preventive measure would be a realistic evaluation of just how far the nuclear reactor program ought to go. The chance of a disaster increases with each added installation. To what extent would the probable benefits of an additional installation justify the increased risk? Significantly enough, the former chairman of the AEC now believes that we have already gone too far in this program.* It is also important to avoid building power reactors near areas which might be involved in an earthquake.

Measures for Minimizing Casualties from Initial Impact

An important safety measure would be to locate all nuclear reactors at a truly safe distance from centers of human habitation. Unfortunately, this is being done only to a limited extent. Most reactors are far enough removed from population centers to give protection against blast; however, safety against radioactive contamination may not be adequate.

Government scientists have estimated the possible consequences of a major accident in a large nuclear power plant. The maximum includes: 3,400 deaths from radiation injury in the surrounding population,

* Lilienthal, D., Whatever Happened to the Peaceful Atom? *Harper's Magazine,* 227: 41, October 1963.

43,000 cases of non-fatal radiation injury, and contamination of 150,000 square miles of land to the extent that restrictions on use of the land for food would be needed.

It should be pointed out, though, that these maximum effects are not likely to occur. Most major accidents would probably produce fewer deaths and injuries than the number listed above. Nevertheless, these figures are useful in giving some indication of the extent of the problem. It is often said that the chance of such a major accident is extremely small because of the safety features in the construction of power reactors. Statements like this have in the past been made in regard to a particular atomic test or an installation, and yet several such accidents have happened. A nuclear power reactor, therefore, must be considered a potential cause of disaster.

Recognition and Warning Signs
None of practical value are known.

Main Mechanisms of Death and Injury
In any future nuclear reactor accidents the main mechanisms of death and injury would be radiation and blast.

Prevention of Further Casualties after Initial Impact
Civil defense monitors should measure radiation levels frequently. If the levels approach the danger point, the public should go to fallout shelters or, if indicated, they should evacuate the area.

Special Procedures and Problems in Rescue, First Aid, Evacuation, and Definitive Medical and Nursing Care
The major problem would be radioactive contamination of the area and of the victims themselves. Radioactive monitoring of the impact area should be carried on continuously to protect the rescue workers. Casualties brought to hospitals should also be monitored and, if necessary, decontaminated. Civil defense personnel may provide useful assistance.

chapter

42 PANIC-CRUSHES

General Description

A panic-crush is a situation in which a panic results in trampling and crushing the victims.

Frequency and Area of Occurrence

Panic-crushes are relatively infrequent, but they can occur whenever large numbers of people are congregated. Usually, they follow or accompany other disasters, increasing the death toll as in the Boston Coconut Grove fire. However, there have been panic-crushes in which many died when no real danger threatened.

In England during World War II, a woman going down wide stairs to an air-raid shelter tripped and screamed. Her scream triggered a panic, and in the rush to get into the shelter about a hundred people were trampled to death. There were no enemy planes in sight, and it is difficult to understand what the people were afraid of. More recently, in Peru, 328 people were killed in a panic-crush during a soccer game when a crowd, trying to avoid police tear-gas, found the exits at the stadium locked. The tear-gas was uncomfortable, but not deadly.

Causes

A major cause of panic-crush is the inherent human tendency to panic under certain circumstances (*see* chapter 4). Another cause, which is readily correctible, consists of inadequate *open* exits from areas where large groups of people are gathered.

Important Past Examples

Most panic-crushes in the past have accompanied other disasters. The only important exception since World War II was the occurence in Peru on May 24, 1964.

Possible Preventive Measures

The most important preventive measures are laws—strictly enforced—requiring adequate, *usable* exits from areas where large numbers of people congregate. The laws should specify the number of exits per 1,000 persons in the area and, further, should provide that they must be kept open while the people are in that area. In the Peruvian disaster, many of the steel gates of the stadium were locked to keep small boys from getting

173

in free. This practice of locking stadium gates after a game is under way is common also in the United States. After most of the spectators are seated, many of the gates are locked and the attendants go to watch the game. The gates are reopened shortly before the game ends. A disaster similar to that in Peru could occur at many an American university football stadium and professional baseball park. The triggering event need not be tear-gas or mob violence. It could be a sudden storm, a minor earthquake or just someone slipping on a stairs or being bitten by a dog and screaming.

A second preventive measure can be taken by persons who understand the basis of panic behavior. If it seems that a panic may develop, an attempt to take charge and restrain the crowd may sometimes be effective.

Measures for Minimizing Casualties from Initial Impact

None are known.

Main Mechanisms of Death and Injury

The crushing and suffocating effects of a pile of bodies are the main mechanisms of death and injury.

Prevention of Further Casualties After Initial Impact

No special measures are known.

Special Procedures and Problems in Rescue, First Aid, Evacuation, and Definitive Medical and Nursing Care

Experience with these disasters is too limited to furnish any information.

43 RAILROAD WRECKS

General Description

A railroad wreck involves a collision, derailment, or other event which suddenly damages or destroys the railroad cars. Passengers may be killed or injured.

Frequency and Area of Occurrence

Minor railroad wrecks occur about every month. Major wrecks, in which 25 or more persons are killed, take place infrequently in the United States. No comparable information is available for other areas of the world. However, foreign railroads are usually less safe than the American ones, as shown by the proportion of the number of dead to the number of passenger miles.

Railroads tend to be the safest method of travel despite the wrecks. However, there is still considerable room for improvement.

Important Past Examples—U.S.A., after World War I

Date	Place	Deaths
February 27, 1921	Porter, Indiana	37
December 5, 1921	Woodmont, Pennsylvania	27
August 5, 1922	Sulphur Springs, Missouri	34
September 27, 1923	Lockett, Wyoming	31
June 16, 1925	Hackettstown, New Jersey	50
September 5, 1926	Waco, Colorado	30
June 19, 1938	Sangus, Montana	47
April 19, 1940	Little Falls, New York	31
July 31, 1940	Cuyahoga Falls, Ohio	43
August 29, 1943	Wayland, New York	27
September 6, 1943	Philadelphia, Pennsylvania	79
December 16, 1943	Rennert, North Carolina	72
July 6, 1944	High Bluff, Tennessee	35
August 4, 1944	Stockton, Georgia	47
September 14, 1944	Dewey, Indiana	29
December 31, 1944	Bagley, Utah	50
August 9, 1945	Michigan, North Dakota	34
April 25, 1946	Naperville, Illinois	45
February 17, 1950	Rockville Center, New York	31
September 11, 1950	Coshocton, Ohio	33
November 22, 1950	Richmond Hill, New York	79

Date	*Place*	*Deaths*
February 6, 1951	Woodbridge, New Jersey	84
January 22, 1956	Los Angeles, California	30
September 15, 1958	Elizabethport, New Jersey	48

Other areas, after World War II

March, 1946	Aracaju, Brazil	185
October, 1946	Madras, India	50
August, 1947	Sumatra	400
April, 1949	South Africa	74
October, 1949	Poland	over 200
November, 1949	South Africa	56
January, 1950	Sirhand, India	54
April, 1950	Rio de Janeiro, Brazil	110
April, 1951	Sakuragicho, Japan	104
June, 1951	Nova Iguacu, Brazil	54
December, 1951	Ceara State, Brazil	53
March, 1952	Rio de Janeiro, Brazil	119
October, 1952	Middlesex, England	112
October, 1953	Sydenham, Australia	50
December, 1953	New Zealand	164
December, 1953	Sakvice, Czechoslovakia	103
January, 1954	Sind Desert, Pakistan	60
February, 1954	Seoul, South Korea	56
September, 1954	Negros Island, Philippines	55
September, 1954	Hyderabad, India	137
September, 1956	Hyderabad, India	121
November, 1956	India	143
September, 1957	Jamaica	175
September, 1957	Pakistan	300
October, 1957	Istanbul, Turkey	89
December, 1957	London, England	89
March, 1958	Rio de Janeiro, Brazil	67
May, 1958	Rio de Janeiro, Brazil	128
May, 1959	Indonesia	140
June, 1959	Rio de Janeiro, Brazil	60

Date	Place	Deaths
June, 1959	Lauffen, Germany	35
May, 1960	Leipzig, Germany	59
November, 1960	Czechoslovakia	110
October, 1961	India	50
December, 1961	Catanzaro, Italy	69
January, 1962	Netherlands	91
February, 1962	Cali, Colombia	40
May, 1962	Tokyo, Japan	163
May, 1962	Voghera, Italy	63
July, 1962	Buxar, India	69
July, 1962	Velars-sur-Ouche, France	40
July, 1962	Rumania	32
October, 1962	Poland	34
November, 1963	Yokohama, Japan	155
January, 1964	Belgrade, Yugoslavia	61
February, 1964	Altamirano, Argentina	70

Causes

Railroad disasters are usually caused by defective equipment, poor management, or bad judgment on the part of operating personnel.

Possible Preventive Measures

A key point in preventing railroad disasters is the recognition that any measures taken should apply to freight trains as well as passenger trains. It would do little good to enforce safety standards for a passenger train if a freight train crashes into it or derails just in front of it.

Frequent safety inspection of all equipment is, of course, vital and is usually carried out properly.

Another important measure is the assignment of at least two men to each locomotive, operating on tracks used by passenger trains. It makes little difference whether the second man is called an assistant engineer, co-engineer, or fireman. His presence may prevent a disaster if the engineer suddenly becomes ill, or ignores a warning signal. Automatic devices, while helpful, are not a complete substitute for a trained person. The stationing of a second person in each locomotive is not "feather-bedding," but an important safety feature.

Some consideration should be given to preventing the type of disaster which occurs when a train, sometimes a freight, is derailed on a track parallel to a passenger track. The derailed cars may not actually be touching the passenger tracks, so that they would not activate automatic block signals. However, they could be close enough to prevent an oncoming train from clearing them. Thus, a speeding passenger train would have no warning until the engineer sighted the wreckage, and then it would be too late. The recent tragedy in Japan occurred when a freight train derailed, and a few minutes later, two crowded passenger trains crashed into it. There are several ways in which this type of accident can be made less likely. One would be the installation of two-way radio sets, similar to the ones used by airplanes, in the engine of each locomotive, including freights. The engineers would report in every ten minutes, and at once if something happened. This would prevent some of the crashes. Even a three-minute warning over the radio could give the engineer of an approaching train time to stop, or to slow down enough to reduce the death toll greatly. If railroads are unwilling to spend money for the safety devices which airplanes have found so useful, a simpler, cheaper method could be tried. Each locomotive and caboose could carry a set of warning rockets which would be sent up at once after a derailment, and at one-minute intervals for at least 30 minutes, or until warning signs have been set out along all approaching tracks.

Measures for Minimizing Casualties from Initial Impact
None are known.

Recognition and Warning Signs
No reliable ones are known.

Main Mechanisms of Death and Injury
Most deaths and injuries are caused by impact or crushing.

Prevention of Further Casualties after Initial Impact
In some railroad disasters, particularly abroad, the deaths and injuries were increased greatly when another train, unaware of the wreck, crashed

into it at a high speed. Therefore, the first action of survivors of a train wreck should be to run along the tracks in both directions for at least a mile, and flag down approaching trains. Between two and six persons should be detailed for this task.

Special Procedures and Problems in Rescue, First Aid, Evacuation, and Definitive Medical and Nursing Care

Since railroad wrecks often take place on stretches of track remote from highways, it may be difficult to reach the area with ordinary vehicles. In such cases, rescue parties should, if possible, proceed to the disaster scene by means of a relief train.

In many wrecks, live victims are trapped in the crushed steel of the railroad cars; special equipment may be needed to free them. It may be necessary to administer plasma to a victim who cannot be freed for some time.

Medical and nursing care do not ordinarily involve any unusual problems.

chapter
44   SHIP DISASTERS

General Description

There are several varieties of ship disaster. Ships may sink in a storm, explode, burn, crash into each other, crash into an iceberg or rock, capsize, or vanish without explanation. Some of the worst ship disasters have taken place in inland waters. We will not consider ship disasters caused by war or those of naval vessels.

Frequency and Area of Occurrence

Major ship disasters take place at irregular intervals. Smaller ones, involving fewer than 100 people, take place several times a year. Ferryboats and excursion boats seem to be particularly dangerous.

Important Past Examples—U. S. Ships, after 1900

Date	Ship	Place	Type	Deaths
Feb. 12, 1907	Larchmont	Long Island	Sinking	131
Nov. 9, 1913	10 ships	Great Lakes	Storm	240
July 24, 1915	Eastland	Chicago River	Capsizing	812
Aug. 16, 1915	San Jacinto-Sam Houston	Gulf of Mexico	Wrecked	106
Oct. 24, 1924	Car Ferry	Milwaukee	Sinking	52
Sept. 8, 1934	Morro Castle	Off New Jersey	Fire	125
Feb. 20, 1963	Marine Sulphur Queen	Atlantic	Unknown	39

Other Ships

April 14, 1912	Titanic (Britain)	Atlantic	Collision with iceberg	1,517
Sept. 28, 1912	Kickermaru (Japan)	Pacific	Sinking	1,000
Oct. 25, 1927	Principessa Mafolda (Italy)	S. Atlantic	Explosion	314
June 14, 1931	St. Philibert (France)	Atlantic	Sinking	450
Feb., 1946	River boat	Nile (Egypt)	Capsizing	50

Date	Ship	Place	Type	Deaths
Mar., 1946	Ferry Kinkazan			
	Maru (Japan)	Pacific	Capsizing	170
Aug., 1946	Vitya	Lake Nyassa		
		(Africa)	Foundering	295
Jan., 1947	Himara (Greece)	Mediterranean	Hit mine	392
Jan., 1947	Chekiang	Pacific	Collision	400
March, 1947	River boat	Yangtze River	Fire	150
June, 1947	River boat	North River		
		(China)	Hit rock	100
July 17, 1947	Ferry (India)	Bombay	Sinking	625
Dec., 1948	Kiangyn (China)	Yangtze River	Explosion	1,172
Sept. 17, 1949	Noronic (Canadian)	Dock	Fire	119
July, 1951	Excursion boat	Spree River		
		(Germany)	Explosion	60
July, 1952	Sailboat			
	(Philippines)	Pacific	Capsizing	50
Sept., 1952	Ferry (Yugoslavia)	Danube River	Capsizing	86
Jan., 1953	Island boat			
	(Philippines)	Pacific	Sinking	80
Jan., 1953	Chang Tyong Ho			
	(Korea)	Pacific	Sinking	244
Jan., 1953	Ferry (Korea)	Pacific	Sinking	53
Feb., 1953	Ferry (Princess			
	Victoria)	Irish Sea	Sinking	132
Feb., 1953	Japanese ship	Pacific	Sinking	67
July, 1953	Ferry (India)	India	Capsizing	60
Sept. 26, 1954	Ferry (Japan)	Strait	Capsizing	1,172
May, 1955	Ferry (Japan)	Inland Sea	Collision	156
June, 1956	Badora (India)	Bengal Bay	Sinking	199
July 25, 1956	Andrea Doria			
	(Italy)	Atlantic	Collision	51
Nov., 1956	Ferry (Formosa)	Pacific	Hit reef	102
April, 1957	River boats (India)	Godavari River	Sinking	150
April, 1957	Ferry (Japan)	Inland Sea	Hit reef	96
May, 1957	River boat (China)	Yangtze River	Fire	100
Oct., 1957	River boat (India)	Assam, India	Capsizing	50
Jan., 1958	Ferry (Japan)	Pacific	Sinking	170
Feb., 1958	Seistan (Britain)	Bahrein	Explosion	53
March, 1958	Ferry	Sea of Marmora	Sinking	350
March, 1958	Ship (unidentified)	Off Java	Sinking	58
March 1, 1958	Ferry (Turkey)	Turkey	Capsizing	361
Oct., 1958	Motor launch			
	(Philippines)	Visayan Sea	Sinking	75

Date	*Ship*	*Place*	*Type*	*Deaths*
Jan. 30, 1959	Hans Hedtoft (Denmark)	Atlantic	Collision with iceberg	95
May, 1959	Dandara (River boat)	Nile	Capsizing	150
June, 1959	Fishing boats (Canadian)	Atlantic	Sinking	35
July, 1959	Motor launch (Denmark)	Atlantic	Explosion	54
March, 1960	Boat	Red Sea	Sinking	50
April, 1960	Motor launch	Persian Gulf	Sinking	57
May, 1960	River boat (India)	Kristna River	Capsizing	100
Jan., 1961	Ship (unidentified)	Off Morocco	Sinking	42
April, 1961	Dara (British)	Persian Gulf	Collision	212
June, 1961	Motor ship (Burma)	Andaman Sea	Sinking	85
July, 1961	Save (Portugal)	Near Mozambique	Explosion	259
Sept., 1961	Tourist boat (Colombia)	Buenaventura Bay	Sinking	74
Oct., 1962	Sanct Sirthun) (Norway)	Off Norway	Ran aground	32
May, 1963	Motor launch (Egypt)	Nile	Capsizing	185
July, 1963	River boat (Argentina)	Plate River	Explosion	53
Dec., 1963	Lakonia (Greece)	Atlantic	Fire	155

Causes

The causes of ship disaster include poor design, improper maintenance, overloading (especially of ferries and excursion boats), poor navigation, bad judgment on the part of officers, and—at times—pure accident. However, analysis of past ship disasters, of which only a small fraction are listed above, indicates that almost all were preventable. A major cause of disaster on ferries and excursion boats has been the congregation of passengers on one side, causing the boat to capsize.

Possible Preventive Measures

The first preventive measure is proper design and construction of ships. This means that more attention should be paid to safety features, and less to extravagant decorations. Apparently, this principle is being followed on the newer American ships which are considered much safer than any of the foreign luxury liners.

Proper maintenance of ships, with elimination of fire and explosion hazards, is important but difficult to enforce on foreign ships.

The vigilance of the U. S. Coast Guard is perhaps the most effective measure in preventing ship disasters. Public support of the Coast Guard is well-deserved.

Measures for Minimizing Casualties from Initial Impact

The most important measure is prior training, and drill of crew and passengers in emergency procedures. Provision of adequate life boats and life rafts is also essential.

Recognition and Warning Signs

Usually, these are technical matters to be handled by the ship's officers and crews. However, the smell of smoke on board a ship is an important warning, and makes it mandatory to notify the captain at once.

Main Mechanisms of Death and Injury

Most deaths come from drowning; others result from fire and explosion.

Prevention of Further Casualties after Initial Impact

This is a matter largely for rescue vessels.

Improvement in the design of life jackets would also save lives. During World War II, and more recently in the Lakonia ship fire, there have been reports of many bodies found floating in life jackets only hours after the disaster. The water was often quite warm, and the cause of death seemed obscure. Reporters described the victims as dying of fright, exposure, exhaustion, or swallowing salt water. All these conditions probably played some role, but in many cases were not the primary cause. Unsatisfactory life jacket design seems an important factor and one which can be corrected.

Most life jackets are designed to keep the person's head above water. This prevents swallowing of water in most cases and allows access to air. However, a victim in a life jacket tends to hang perpendicularly; his diaphragm and abdominal muscles are below the surface of the water. Under normal physiological conditions, the diaphragm and other respiratory muscles move air into and out of the lungs without working against any significant pressure differences. Respiratory muscles are relatively thin, weak muscles, and when they are submerged, it means that with every liter of air inhaled a liter of water has to be pushed away. The work load involved, therefore, even in quiet breathing becomes much, much greater than when the body is not immersed in water. As a result, the person in a standard life jacket soon exhausts his respiratory muscles and dies of suffocation unless he is rescued promptly. Toward the end, he may thrash around and swallow some water, thus hastening his death. Some persons with exceptionally powerful respiratory muscles—trained athletes, for example—can survive for more than a day in such circumstances, but not the average victim of a ship disaster.

The remedy for this problem may be fairly simple. Life preservers should be redesigned so that in addition to keeping the head above water, they also keep at least part of the diaphragm above water. It may help to change the position of the victim from a perpendicular one to a position nearly parallel to the surface, such as is used in the back-float.

Special Procedures and Problems in Rescue, First Aid, Evacuation, and Definitive Medical and Nursing Care

The Coast Guard and nearby ships handle the rescue, first aid, and evacuation. Usually, the survivors do not require much specialized care, unless there have been serious burns. (*See* chapter 33.)

45 TORNADOES

General Description

Tornadoes are rotary storms of the highest intensity but of the smallest area. Winds in a tornado rotate counterclockwise, with rotary wind speeds over 200 miles per hour —perhaps as high as 500 miles per hour. There is usually a heavy rain; there is also a characteristic funnel cloud, and a roaring sound.

The entire tornado funnel moves forward at moderate speeds, averaging 35 to 40 miles per hour. The maximum forward speed of the funnel is about 70 miles per hour. The width of a tornado funnel ranges from 10 yards to a mile, with an average of about 400 yards. The length of a tornado track ranges from a few yards to 200 miles, with an average of 16 miles. The average duration of a tornado is less than one hour. The most persistent one on record lasted seven hours. Tornadoes kill an average of 222 Americans each year, and injure about 2,000.

Frequency and Area of Occurrence

In the United States, there are several hundred tornadoes per year, but fortunately only a few cause major injuries or death. The incidence is lowest in January, begins to rise in February, reaches a peak in June, and then gradually becomes lower again. The initial areas involved are usually the south-central plains of Texas. Then the incidence moves gradually northward with the spring and summer months. Usually, tornadoes track from the southwest to the northeast. The usual time for a tornado to strike is between noon and midnight. It has happened that several tornadoes have occurred on the same day in the same general area. Despite our knowledge of the *average* or *usual* pattern of a tornado, we must remember that a tornado can strike any part of the country, at any time, and can follow any path. Some of the most destructive tornadoes have occurred outside the so-called tornado belt.

It is particularly important to realize that a ring of hills around an area does *not* protect it from a tornado, despite popular belief. Some of the worst hit areas, such as Worcester, Massachusetts, have had a ring of hills on the side from which the tornado came.

Important Past Examples—U.S.A., after 1925

Date	Place	Deaths
March 18, 1925	Missouri, Illinois, Indiana	689
March 21, 1932	Alabama	268
April 5, 1936	Tupelo, Mississippi	216
April 6, 1936	Gainesville, Georgia	203
June 23, 1944	Ohio, Pennsylvania, W. Virginia, and Maryland	150
April 12, 1945	Oklahoma and Arkansas	102
April 9, 1947	Texas, Oklahoma, and Kansas	169
March 21, 22, 1952	Arkansas, Missouri, and Tennessee	208
May 11, 1953	Waco, Texas	114
June 8, 1953	Flint, Michigan	116
June 9, 1953	Worcester, Massachusetts	90
May 5, 1960	Oklahoma and Arkansas	29

Note: This series contains two sets of tornadoes, striking—a day apart—first a midwestern and then an eastern area. In 1917, a similar pair was noted. This is not likely to be mere coincidence. It suggests that the disturbance causing the tornado dipped down in a midwestern area, then raised up so that no funnel was visible, continued in an easterly direction for a day and then dipped down again. Accordingly, if a midwestern area has been struck by a major tornado, the eastern part of the nation should be on the alert for one during the next day or two.

Other Areas: records of tornadoes in other nations are incomplete.

Causes

The exact causes of a tornado are not known. They are probably related to situations in which a layer of heavy, cold air rests on top of a layer of light, warm air.

Possible Preventive Measures

None are known at this time.

Measures for Minimizing Initial Casualties

Tornado shelters have been life-savers in the past. A warning network would be of great value, as well as better training of the population in protective measures. Stronger construction of schools, with tornado-proof areas, seems important. (Several schools have been destroyed by tornadoes, and many children were killed and injured.) Until stronger schools are available, school children should be sent home whenever the weather bureau reports that tornadoes are likely to occur in a particular area. Even an ordinary home basement-corner is safer in a tornado than most schools. Plans for stronger school buildings are available.

In general, the southwest corner of a basement is the safest part of a home during a tornado; it is safer than being out of doors. If caught out of doors, however, it is usually safest to lie flat in a shallow ditch or depression.

Recognition and Warning Signs

Early warning of a tornado can often be obtained by the weather bureau through radar. Such warning can then be broadcast to the public by radio and television.

A probable indication of a tornado is a heavy cloud formation in which the clouds seem to be moving in all directions at once, rather than in a single major direction. Large hailstones are said to signify tornado conditions, but we have no data on the reliability of this sign.

An absolute sign of a tornado is the sighting of a funnel cloud. It can often be seen far enough away to allow people to get to shelter.

When the tornado is quite close, it sounds like an express train overhead—and then there are usually only a few seconds left before it strikes.

Main Mechanisms of Death and Injury

The winds of a tornado exert forces which are difficult to comprehend. The force produced by wind increases roughly according to the square of the velocity. Thus, a wind of 40 miles per hour exerts a force which is four times as great as a wind of 20 miles per hour. A wind of 50 miles per hour will usually knock down many pedestrians; a wind of 200 miles per hour (which is not unusual for a tornado) exerts 4x4 or 16 times the force of a 50 miles per hour wind. A wind of 500 miles per hour, which some experts believe occurs in tornadoes, exerts a force *100 times* as great as a 50 miles per hour wind.

Tornadoes blow heavy refrigerators out of houses; automobiles have been blown off the roads and hundreds of yards into the air; railroad cars have been blown completely off the tracks; wood planks have been driven through large tree trunks.

In addition to the blowing force exerted by the tornado, there is a suction phase in which the atmospheric pressure drops by as much as two pounds per square inch (288 pounds per square foot). Floor construction in private homes is based on ability to stand 40-pounds-per-square-foot pressure differentials; walls and ceilings are even weaker. Therefore, when the suction phase of a tornado strikes a house, the entire structure tends to blow outward and people and furniture are lifted into the air.

There is a 1-2-3 pattern to the impact of a tornado. First, there are the high winds, then there is the suction phase, and finally, the high winds return.

People are injured or killed by being hit by flying debris, by being smashed against buildings, trees or the ground, or by a combination of all these factors.

Prevention of Further Casualties after Initial Impact

The most important step if a tornado strikes a heavily populated area is the prevention of fire. Although a heavy rain accompanies most tornadoes, it is of too short a duration to soak into most of the lumber used in home construction. This lumber is, therefore, still quite inflammable. It is scattered all around after a tornado. Gas lines are usually broken, and escaping gas adds to the fire danger. Electric wires are usually down, and short circuits can provide the sparks to start fires. If fires start and are not controlled, they could develop into a mass conflagration, killing all the injured and some of the rescuers.

Therefore, all electric power to the area should be turned off, immediately after a tornado has struck, by the first man in the power plant who can reach the switch, and gas should also be turned off at once.

Firemen should first concentrate on stopping and preventing fires—a task which should receive absolute top priority.

Secondly, a watch should be kept for another tornado in the same general area. After the initial tornado impact, the number of people in the area will soon have increased about ten times; if a second tornado strikes nearby without warning, the casualties, also, would be ten times as great.

Special Procedures and Problems in Rescue, First Aid, Evacuation, and Definitive Medical and Nursing Care

After a tornado, victims can be found in all sorts of unusual places—blown into fields, on top of roofs, and under debris. Therefore, rescue efforts should include a thorough search of the area, including a margin of at least 100 yards on either side of the tornado track.

In rescuing the injured from under piles of debris, care should be taken to shore up the debris so that it does not collapse on the victims and rescuers, killing and injuring still more.

First-aid procedures are essential before evacuation, as in most other disasters. In evacuating the injured, the usual considerations of avoiding speed and rough driving apply.

A factor affecting definitive medical care is the markedly dirty state of most of the injured. The tornado winds often plaster the victims with mud. Before the extent of an injury can be determined, it usually must be washed carefully. Accordingly, some provisions should be made for cleaning the mud from the casualties as gently and efficiently as possible.

In addition, all tornado-caused lacerations must be considered to be grossly contaminated. Experience has shown that they cannot safely be sutured on the assumption that they are clean wounds. To be sure, by the time the victims arrive in the operating room, the wounds may have been washed enough so that, superficially, they look clean. However, they are still contaminated, and primary suturing is contra-indicated.

46   TSUNAMIS (TIDAL WAVES, SEISMIC WAVES)

General Description

A tsunami is an ocean wave caused by an earthquake in the floor of the ocean. The term "tidal wave" is misleading, since a tsunami has nothing to do with the tides. However, it should be used in giving warning.

Tsunamis travel at speeds of about 400 miles per hour, and can move from one end of an ocean to the other. The tsunami of April 1, 1946, traveled 8,000 miles through the Pacific. On the open seas, the tsunami is not ordinarily visible, since the crest-to-crest distance is many miles— up to 100— and since much of the wave energy is transmitted in the form of a low, very wide wave. However, when a tsunami reaches a sloping shore, the water in it begins to pile up into an enormous wave which looks like a solid wall of water. Tsunami waves over 50 feet high have been reported. Furthermore, the speed of the wave is such that enormous amounts of energy are contained within it.

Frequency and Area of Occurrence

Tsunamis large enough to cause injury or death occur once every few years. They are most common on the borders and islands of the Pacific and Indian oceans. However, all coasts are susceptible to them.

Important Past Examples—U.S.A.

Date	Place	Deaths
May 23, 24, 1960	Hawaii (also Japan and Okinawa)	237

Other Areas:

November 1, 1755	Lisbon, Portugal (+ earthquake)	60,000
November 18, 1929	Newfoundland	27
November 6, 1942	Bengal, India	10,000
October 10, 1960	East Pakistan	6,000
October 31, 1960	East Pakistan	4,000

Causes

Tsunamis are caused by earthquakes on the ocean floor or near the coast.

Possible Preventive Measures

No preventive measures are known.

Measures for Minimizing Casualties from Initial Impact

Improvement in seismographic analysis of earthquakes on the ocean floor to provide an adequate warning period would be the most important protective measure.

Teaching as many people as possible the usual signs of an impending tsunami (*see* below) would help reduce casualties.

Setting up loud-speakers or other warning systems on public beaches to spread news of an impending tsunami rapidly might also be worthwhile.

Immediate evacuation of beaches and low-lying areas on receiving warning of a possible tsunami is essential. The evacuation should be as complete as possible; merely running back to the boardwalk area or just beyond would not be sufficient. Large ships have been carried by tsunamis well beyond such areas. In general, it is advisable to keep moving away from the ocean as rapidly as possible, until at least one mile from the shore, or until an elevation of 150 feet above sea level is reached. Man-made structures, no matter how substantial looking, do not protect against tsunamis.

Recognition and Warning Signs

The sub-ocean quake which gives rise to a tsunami *may* be recorded and accurately identified by seismographs in time. There may be an interval of several hours after the quake occurs until the tsunami strikes the coast. In that case, adequate warning can be given. However, it is not yet certain that our seismographic techniques and apparatus are effective enough, or the instruments manned sufficiently to provide such a timely warning in all cases.

In some cases, depending on the type of beach, the water will suddenly recede below the usual low-tide line a few minutes before the tsunami strikes. Tragically, in some past episodes, the significance of the receding ocean was not understood by the people on the shore and they walked out to look at the ocean bottom. When they saw the great wave coming, it was too late to save themselves. Whenever the water level at an ocean beach becomes lowered rapidly, it should be assumed that a tsunami will strike in a few minutes, and everyone should run—not walk —away from the water. It is virtual suicide to remain on the beach, waiting to see the tsunami. By the time it is sighted, it will be traveling about 400 miles per hour, so that there won't be time to take more than a few steps.

Main Mechanisms of Death and Injury

Drowning, and crushing by debris carried along by the water at high speeds, are the main causes of death and injury.

Prevention of Further Casualties after Initial Impact

The likelihood of multiple tsunamis must always be kept in mind. In the tsunamis of May 1960, the third and fourth waves striking the Chilean coast were higher than the first or second in some places. Many people died because they returned to the coast too quickly. In the rather small tsunami which struck Crescent City, California, after the Alaska earthquake of March 27, 1964, it was the fourth wave which caused all the deaths and most of the damage. Therefore, it is vital to keep crowds away from the impact area. First-aid workers must themselves be alert to possible multiple waves and avoid the unnecessary loss of their own lives.

Special Procedures and Problems in Rescue, First Aid, Evacuation, and Definitive Medical and Nursing Care

In this type of disaster, no special procedures or problems have been reported. In part, this may be due to the fact that a very high proportion of the casualties are deaths.

Special Note

As pointed out above, tsunamis have been quite rare on the Atlantic coast, compared to the Pacific. However, they may occur. Despite their rarity, they are a great menace because of the potential deaths they could cause. If a tsunami were to strike the Atlantic coast of the United States without warning on an afternoon in July or August, it might well kill several million persons—more than all the other disasters in our nation's history put together. In this case, the low probability of occurrence is more than balanced by the potential death rate. Accordingly, a sound disaster-prevention philosophy suggests that our seismographic facilities be improved, and that they be manned 24 hours a day on the Atlantic as well as Pacific coast, so that warning of a possible tsunami can be given in time.

47 VOLCANIC ERUPTIONS

General Description

A volcanic eruption is an outpouring of molten rock (lava) from an opening in the earth's crust. At times, the liquid rock may ooze out slowly; at other times it may be blown out with explosive force. In many cases, ashes and poisonous gases are ejected with the lava. The lava cools fairly rapidly into a solid rock, and layer upon layer is built up to produce a volcanic cone or mountain. Such mountains are being formed all the time. In 1943, a new one, Paricutin, developed in a cornfield in Mexico. In most cases, volcanic eruptions occur at the sites of pre-existing volcanic cones— an area which already contains cracks in the earth's crust. When a large amount of lava and other material is blown out of a volcano with great force near a populated area, it produces a disaster. Some volcanoes have been described as extinct, meaning that they can no longer produce eruptions; others have been called dormant, meaning that they are not actually pouring out lava or smoke but might do so sometime in the future. Sometimes, a volcano has been considered dormant or extinct for 1,000 years, and then has suddenly erupted. This occurred in Bandai-San in Japan in 1888.

Frequency and Area of Occurrence

Volcanic eruptions producing disasters are not common. However, when they occur, the loss of life can be great. Most active volcanoes are found in certain areas of the world. The islands of Hawaii are volcanic in origin and have a number of active volcanoes. Several volcanoes in the continental United States are dormant, or believed to be extinct. They include Mts. Rainier and Baker in Washington, Mts. Shasta and Lassen Peak in California, and Mt. Hood in Oregon. Mts. Baker and Lassen Peak have been active within the past 150 years.

Important Past Examples—Other Areas

Date	Place	Deaths
August 24, 79 A.D.	Mt. Vesuvius (Pompeii)	20,000
August 27, 1883	Krakatoa (East Indies)	35,000 (most in a tsunami)

Date	Place	Deaths
July 15, 1888	Bandai-San, Japan	460
May 8, 1902	Mount Pelee, Martinique	40,000
March 17, 1963	Bali	1,500
March 3, 1964	Conaripe, Chile	over 25

Causes

Volcanic eruptions are caused by molten gaseous materials escaping from a gap in the earth's crust.

Possible Preventive Measures

None are known.

Measures for Minimizing Casualties from Initial Impact

Warning signs must be heeded and evacuation carried out promptly. Part of the tragedy of some past disasters is that the volcanoes gave ample warning that something was coming, yet little was done about it. The worst example was the Mt. Pelee eruption in 1902. For many years, the volcano had been dormant. Then in April, 1902, smoke and ashes were discharged. On May 2, there were loud explosions and the people became alarmed. The governor of Martinique, with the help of a commission, reassured the people and told them there was no need to flee. Then on the morning of May 8, the main eruption took place, killing every inhabitant of the city of St. Pierre, except for a condemned prisoner in a deep stone dungeon. If the people had been somewhat more fearful, or the governor less "brave," they would have survived.

The historic eruption of Mt. Vesuvius which destroyed Pompeii also gave several days warning, and those who heeded it survived.

Recognition and Warning Signs

The escape of smoke (really fine dust at a high temperature) or other material from a volcano is a general warning. If the volcano had been considered dormant or extinct, any increase in its activity should be considered ominous.

Main Mechanisms of Death and Injury

Most victims of a volcanic eruption are killed by poisonous fumes, superheated gases, or masses of volcanic dust. The inhabitants of Pompeii are believed to have been smothered under a 10 to 14 foot thick layer of volcanic dust which fell on them.

Prevention of Further Casualties after Initial Impact

Evacuate all survivers, and keep all other persons away from the area in case another eruption takes place.

Special Procedures and Problems in Rescue, First Aid, Evacuation, and Definitive Medical and Nursing Care

The major problem would be evacuation of survivors without endangering the rescuers. Special types of vehicles and oxygen masks may be needed.

There have been so few survivors of these eruptions that we have little or no experience for future guidance.

Bibliography

Airplane Crashes
Civil Aeronautics Board. *Statistical Review and Resume of Accidents—Calendar Year 1961,* Washington, D. C., 1964.

Avalanches
McDowell, B. and Fletcher, J. E. Avalanche! 3,500 Peruvians Perish in Seven Minutes. *National Geographic, 121*:855, 1962.

Earthquakes
Bronson, W. *The Earth Shook, the Sky Burned.* Doubleday, Garden City, N. Y., 1959.
Chick, A. C. *Transactions.* Am. Geophysical Union, Washington, D. C., 1933.
Fuller, M. L. *The New Madrid Earthquake.* U. S. Geological Survey, Bulletin 494, Washington, D. C., 1912.
Hodgson, J. H. *Earthquakes and Earth Structure.* Prentice-Hall, Englewood Cliffs, N. J. 1964.
Leet, L. D. Earthquakes. *Ann. Amer. Acad. Pol. and Soc. Sci., 309*:36, Ja. 1957.
Matthews, S. W. The Night the Mountain Moved. *National Geographic, 117*: 328, March 1960.
Saidi, F. The 1962 Earthquake in Iran. *New Eng. J. Med., 268*:929, 1963.
Walsh, J. Alaska: A Thorough Postmortem on Earthquake Urged on Behalf of Both Science, Reconstruction. *Science, 144*:515, 1964.

Epidemics
Creighton, C. *A History of Epidemics in Britain.* Cambridge University Press, Cambridge, 1891.
Gasquet, F. A. *The Black Death of 1348 and 1349.* Geo. Bell and Sons, London, 1908.
Gill, C. A. *The Genesis of Epidemics.* William Wood, Baltimore, 1928.
Hecker, J. F. C. *Epidemics of the Middle Ages.* Woodfall Publications, London, 1844.
Mullett, C. F. *The Bubonic Plague and England.* U. of Kentucky Press, Lexington, 1956.
Prinzing, F. *Epidemics Resulting from Wars.* Clarendon Press, Oxford, 1916.
Report of Epidemic Commission of the League of Nations. Geneva, 1921.
Scientific American, 105:169, August 19, 1911.
Smith, G. *Plague on Us.* Oxford University Press, New York, 1943.

Surgeon-General's Office, War Department. *Cholera Epidemic of 1873 in the United States.* U. S. Government Printing Office, Washington, D. C., 1875.

U.S.A.F. *Studies With a Simulated Martian Environment: Bacterial Survival and Soil Moisture Content.* School of Aerospace Medicine, Brooks A. F. Base, Texas, Nov. 1962.

Winslow, C. E. A. *Man and Epidemics.* Princeton U. Press, Princeton, N. J. Princeton, N. J., 1943.

Winslow, C. E. A. *Man and Epidemics.* Princeton U. Press, Princeton, N. J., 1952.

Zinsser, H. *Rats, Lice and History.* Little, Brown, Boston, 1935.

Explosions

Blocker, V. and Blocker, T. G., Jr. The Texas City Disaster. *Am. J. Surg.,* 78: 756, 1949.

The Los Angeles Explosion. *Disaster,* 1:12, 1947.

Fires, General

Building Exits Code. 19th ed., National Fire Protection Association, Boston.

Building Materials List. Underwriters Laboratories, Inc., Chicago, 1962.

Dominge, C. C. and Lincoln, W. O. *Building Construction as Applied to Fire Insurance.* 4th ed., Chilton, Philadelphia, 1949.

Downey, F. The First Great Fire in Red Cross History. *Disaster,* 1:8, 1947.

Editorial: Fire. *Disaster,* 1:3, 1947.

Fire Safe School Buildings. National Board of Fire Underwriters, New York, N. Y.

Kearney, P. W. *Disaster on Your Doorstep.* Harper, New York, 1953.

Moore, F. D. The Treatment of Severe Burns. *Am. J. of Nursing,* 54:454, 1954.

National Building Code. National Board of Fire Underwriters, New York, N. Y.

National Fire Codes. National Fire Protection Association, Boston, 1962.

Redmond, J. H. Industry Defense Preparedness Pays Off in Peacetime Emergencies. *Industrial Security,* 6:105, 1962.

Standard for Installation of Centrifugal Fire Pumps. National Fire Protection Association, Boston, 1961.

Standard for Installation of Sprinkler Systems. National Fire Protection Association, Boston, 1961.

A Study of Fire Problems. National Research Council, Publication 949, Washington, D. C., 1961.

Wallace, D. B. The Industrial Fire Brigade in a Civil Defense Emergency. *Industrial Security,* 6:48, 1962.

Fires, Hospitals

Babcock, C. I. A Place for Old Folks to Live: Fire Safety in the Nursing Home, I. *Hospital Management*, 85:48, Jan. 1958.

Babcock, C. I. A Place for Old Folks to Live: Fire Safety in the Nursing Home, II. *Hospital Management*, 85:47, Feb. 1958.

Barton, J. In Case of Fire: Minutes Mean Lives. *Modern Hospital*, 83:5, Nov. 1954.

Booth, G. W. Hospital Fires. *Disaster, 3,* Sept., Oct. 1949.

Guidelines to Hospital Fire Safety. *Hospitals; J.A.H.A.,* Special Issue, June 1, 1962.

Fires, Schools

Buehring, L. E. Simulated Horror Taught: Evacuation in Mock School Fire. *The Nation's Schools,* 64:53, 1959.

Building Exits Code. 13th ed., National Fire Protection Association, Boston, 1956.

Checklist of Safety Education in Your School. National Education Association, Washington, D. C.

Crosby, E. U. et al. *N.F.P.A. Handbook of Fire Protection.* 11th ed., National Fire Protection Association, Boston, 1954.

Finchum, R. N. and Boerrigter, G. C. *School Fires: Prevention, Control, Protection.* Department of Health, Education, and Welfare, Washington, D. C., 1962.

Fire Exit Drill Signalling Devices and Fire Drill Regulations. National Safety Council, Chicago, Ill.

Fire Safe School Buildings. National Board of Fire Underwriters, New York, N. Y.

Garber, L. O. Abate the Fire Hazard. *The Nation's Schools,* 63:57, 1959.

How Safe Are the Schools? *U. S. News and World Report,* December 12, 1958.

Is Your Student Housing Fire Safe? Federation of Mutual Fire Insurance Companies, Chicago, Ill.

Laboratories-Fire Record Bulletin FR 58-3. National Fire Protection Association, Boston, Mass.

Reasons, G. Smoke is the Killer. *The Nation's Schools,* 64:61, 1959.

School Fires. Data Sheet No. 47. National Safety Council, Chicago, Ill.

Floods

Heiser, V. Just Short of Eternity. *Disaster, 1:2,* 1947.

Instituut voor Sociaal Onderzoek van het Nederlandse Volk. *Studies in Holland Flood Disaster in 1953.* By the Instituut and the Committee on Disaster Studies of the National Academy of Sciences —National Research Council, Washington, D. C. The Hague, 1955, 4 vols.

Lemons, H. Physical Characteristics of Disaster: Historical and Statistical Review. *Ann. Amer. Acad. Pol. and Soc. Sci.,* 309:1, Jan. 1957.
Leopold, L. B. and Langbein, W. B. *A Primer on Water, 1960.* Superintendent of Documents, U. S. Government Printing Office, Washington 25, D. C.
Stiles, W. W. How A Community Met a Disaster: Yuba City Flood, December 1955. *Ann. Amer. Acad. Pol. and Soc. Sci.,* 309:160, Jan. 1957.
Sturgis, S. D., Jr. Floods. *Ann. Amer. Acad. Pol. and Soc. Sci.,* 309:15, Jan. 1957.
Tennessee Valley Authority. *Flood Damage Prevention, an Indexed Bibliography.* Knoxville, 1963.

Highway Accidents
Automobile Seat Belts. Report of Special Subcommittee on Traffic Safety. House of Representatives, Aug. 30, 1957. U. S. Government Printing Office, Washington, D. C.
Campbell, H. E. Seat Belts, *J.A.M.A.,* March 11, 1961.
Editorial: Safety Last. *Canadian Med. Assn. Journal,* 72:378, 1955.
Lake, A. Cars Can Be Crash-Proof. *New York Herald Tribune,* Mar. 6, 1955, Section 7, p. 7.
Research Needs in Traffic Safety. Hearing Before a Subcommittee of the Committee on Interstate and Foreign Commerce. House of Representatives, April 23, 1958. U. S. Government Printing Office, Washington, D. C.
Shelden, C. H. Prevention, The Only Cure for Head Injuries Resulting from Automobile Accidents. *J. A. M. A., 159:*981, 1955.

Hurricanes
Battan, L. J. *The Nature of Violent Storms.* Doubleday, Garden City, N. Y., 1961.
Harris, D. L. *Characteristics of the Hurricane Storm Surge.* Technical Paper #48, Department of Commerce, U. S. Weather Bureau, Washington, D. C., 1963.
Reichelderfer, F. W. Hurricanes, Tornadoes, and Other Storms. *Ann. Amer. Acad. Pol. and Soc. Sci.,* 309:23, 1957.

Mine Disasters
Beach, H. D. and Lucas, R. A., eds. *Individual and Group Behavior in a Coal Mine Disaster.* Disaster Study Number 13. National Academy of Sciences—National Research Council, Publication 834, Washington, D. C., 1961.
Forbes, J. J., Ankeny, M. J. and Feehan, F. *Coal Miner's Safety Manual.* U. S. Government Printing Office, Washington, D. C., 1943.

Nuclear Reactor Accidents

Hayes, D. F. *A Summary of Accidents and Incidents Involving Radiation in Atomic Energy Activities, June 1945 through December 1955.* Atomic Energy Commission, Washington, D. C., 1956.

Smith, R. J. *Reactor Safety.* A Literature Search. U. S. Atomic Energy Commission, Washington, D. C., March 1963.

Tornadoes

Form, W. H. and Nosow, S. *Community in Disaster.* Harper, New York, 1958.

Moore, H. E. *Tornadoes Over Texas.* U. of Texas Press, Austin, 1958.

Our Shelter From the Stormy Blast. *Disaster* 4:3, Apr. 1950.

Perry, S. E., Silber, E. and Block, D. A. *The Child and His Family in Disaster: A Study of the 1953 Vicksburg Tornado.* Disaster Study Number 5. National Academy of Sciences—National Research Council, Publication 394, Washington, D. C., 1956.

Tsunamis

Carson, R. *The Sea Around Us.* Oxford University Press, New York, 1951.

Natural Disasters. Navdocks, P-88, Department of the Navy, Washington, D. C., 1961.

Volcanic Eruptions

Maiuri, A., Bianchi, P. V. and Battaglia, L. E. Last Moments of the Pompeians. *National Geographic, 120*:651, 1961.

Wheeler, P. J. F. Death of an Island, Tristan da Cunha. *National Geographic, 121*:678, 1962.

THERMONUCLEAR DISASTER

A thermonuclear war would produce a disaster of the greatest magnitude, comparable only to the great plagues of the Middle Ages. Because of the large areas and the numbers of persons involved, the principles and solutions which apply to lesser disasters cannot be relied upon in thermonuclear disasters without critical examination.

The most important modifying factor in a thermonuclear war would be the presence of radioactive fallout. This would modify all plans for rescue and first aid as described in chapter 52.

In an ordinary disaster, the number of casualties is small in relation to the total population and the resources of the nation. Shortage of vital personnel or materials seldom lasts for more than a day, and usually, there is a surplus of almost everything. On the other hand, in a thermonuclear disaster the total number of casualties would be high in relation to population and resources; therefore, there would be a severe shortage of personnel and supplies.

Studies of lesser disasters have shown that prior planning and preparation could reduce the number of dead and injured considerably. Similarly, studies of thermonuclear weapons effects have shown—clearly and decisively—that prior planning and preparation could greatly reduce the casualty rate. Some indication of the extent to which the death rate from a thermonuclear attack would be reduced can be obtained from Fig. 7. Nevertheless, it should be clear to everybody that, even with the best possible protection, such an attack would result in a large number of casualties.

Many people are unwilling to consider the possibility of a thermonuclear war. They call it "unthinkable" and for them it is. However, for those who have responsibilities for the survival of others—and the nation—every possi-

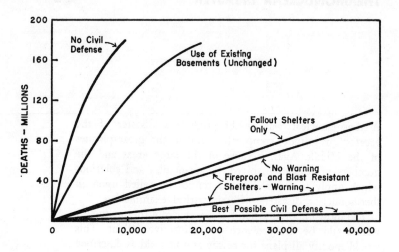

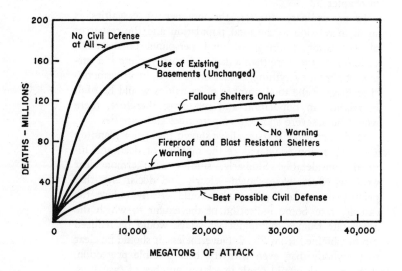

Fig. 7. Estimate of death rate in various shelters from enemy attack directed (top) primarily at military targets, and (bottom) primarily at cities.

bility, however grim and distasteful, is worth being considered rationally and calmly.

In the discussion of the lesser disasters we emphasized disaster prevention as the best possible solution. This applies even more strongly to thermonuclear war. Everything possible—short of surrender—should be tried to lessen the threat of this type of disaster. The American government has consistently striven to find an honorable and peaceful solution to the world's problems. We may be sure that it will continue to do so. Whenever possible, individual citizens should help—and in many cases they do—by joining such agencies as the Peace Corps. However, hasty and over-emotional responses to international tensions on the part of citizens do not help and may hinder our efforts to insure peace.

It should be obvious that the final decision on whether there will be peace or war may not rest with the American government or the public, but with an adversary determined to destroy us. If he orders a thermonuclear attack on our nation, a reasonable civil defense system could save tens of millions of lives. The question has been raised whether civil defense increases in some measure the likelihood of war. The answer has been carefully worked out: civil defense does not increase the risk of war. If anything, it decreases the risk of one type of attack—that of a premeditated sneak attack. Some fears have been expressed that a good civil defense program might make an American president more reckless. This seems extremely unlikely. No one suggests that the presence of lifeboats on a ship makes the captain more reckless. Perhaps the best evidence of the compatibility of civil defense and efforts to remain at peace comes from the example of two countries: the best civil defense programs in the world, by a great margin, are those of Sweden and Switzerland, the most peaceful nations on earth; Sweden has not been at war since Napoleon's time, and Switzerland has been at peace for an even longer period.

Sometimes, one hears the suggestion that the energy and efforts that go into civil defense should instead be channeled into efforts to promote peace. Superficially, this may sound attractive, but when one asks how the energies devoted to civil defense can be transformed into effective means to insure peace, no sensible answer is forthcoming.

Recommendations for measures that help minimize loss of life in other disasters seldom provoke much opposition. By contrast, civil defense proposals have called forth a great deal of vociferous opposition, some even from educated and learned persons. It is important to keep this opposition in perspective and not to be misled by the arguments offered.

For several years completely erroneous stories about firestorm hazards were widely circulated in an effort to discredit civil defense planning. It took a long time to catch up with these errors. Chapter 50 has been included to clarify this area. Those opposed to civil defense have raised dozens of arguments against it, some of them mutually contradictory, and most of them based on technical inaccuracies. It is not within the scope of this book to refute each of these arguments. Others have done that, however, and the interested reader is referred to the topical bibliography at the end of this section for a more detailed discussion.

Those who are satisfied with a less detailed investigation of civil defense pros and cons, may be satisfied with the judgment of persons whose record of positive service to mankind is well-known. Among organizations endorsing the principle of an effective civil defense program are the following:

The American Hospital Association
The Red Cross
The American Medical Association
The AFL-CIO
The Salvation Army.

The Salvation Army has taken an even more positive and effective step than simply endorsing civil defense: it has sent more than 400 of its officers to take special civil defense courses. The National League for Nursing is working with the office of civil defense in studying the relation of nurses and nursing to the total civil defense effort.

It should be noted that endorsement of the principle of civil defense does not necessarily mean complete agreement on every detail. There are still questions about the relative effectiveness of different civil defense measures and constructive criticism is to be welcomed. The concepts of civil defense are not static. They change with the nature of the threat, distribution and training of the American public, new research findings, and with the development of new active defense measures. However, reliance upon shelters will probably remain a primary factor.

48 NUCLEAR RADIATION

Nuclear radiation is rather unfamiliar to most people. Although it would be helpful to understand the basic physics behind nuclear radiation, it is not feasible to include such material in this book. Instead, this chapter will be limited to those aspects which must be understood in order to plan intelligently for personal, family, community, and national survival.

Types of Radiation

The types of radiation which will be discussed are alpha particles, beta particles, gamma rays, and neutrons.

Alpha particles—Alpha particles are the same as the nuclei of helium atoms. They have a relatively high mass and electrical charge and very poor powers of penetration, compared with other forms of radiation. A few inches of air, a layer of clothing, or even the outer layer of skin, can stop them. Therefore, alpha particles *outside* the body are not dangerous. However, if they are emitted inside the body, from swallowed or inhaled fallout, they are about 20 times as damaging as the same amount of gamma rays. Ordinary Geiger counters and radiation survey meters do not pick up alpha particles. Special instruments would be needed for this purpose. But since alpha particles emanate from the same fallout material as gamma rays, the intensity of the gamma radiation can be used as a rough but serviceable guide to the intensity of alpha radiation.

Beta particles—Beta particles are electrons. They are somewhat more penetrating than alpha particles. A few feet of air or several layers of clothing are needed to block them. If they emanate from materials on the skin, they can cause serious burns. Therefore, it is important to wash all fallout particles from the skin. Beta rays emanating from swallowed or inhaled particles are slightly more damaging than gamma rays but less damaging than alpha particles. Special instruments are needed to measure beta radiation. For a rough guide, one may consider the beta radiation to be proportional to the gamma radiation for fallout particles.

Gamma rays—Gamma rays are high-frequency electromagnetic radiations. They resemble X-rays but have a higher frequency and much greater penetrating power. They can travel through several miles of air and through several feet of wood. They can be picked up and counted by several types of measuring instruments. The major radiation danger comes from gamma rays. There are different kinds of gamma rays with different degrees of penetrating power. Gamma rays cannot induce radioactivity in materials which they strike.

Neutrons—Neutrons are particles without electric charge, found in atomic nuclei. They can penetrate substantial thicknesses of most materials. When they hit nuclei of certain atoms, they can knock out other neutrons, just as a billiard ball can transmit its energy to another billiard ball. Therefore, even a thick layer of steel may not give adequate protection from neutrons. But concrete and earth, because of their chemical natures, do offer protection. The mechanism is complex and need not be discussed here. Neutrons can induce radioactivity in materials which they strike. *However, neutrons are not given off by fallout particles.*

Therefore, fallout particles that land on food or water containers do not contaminate the contents. Neutrons radiate from the fireball of a thermonuclear detonation. They have an effective range of about two to three miles in air. Therefore, food and water found within three miles of the fireball should not be consumed, even if it was stored in a closed container—unless it was covered by five feet of earth or three-and-one-half feet of concrete.

A neutron bomb is a theoretical contrivance which releases large amounts of neutrons but no blast, heat, or fallout. It could kill everything within three miles, even in most shelters. However, this is so much less than the lethal range of a hydrogen bomb of equal size (*see* Table II, p. 212) that no nation has as yet bothered to make one. Neutron bombs do not make fallout shelters obsolete—they would make them unnecessary if an adversary were gentle enough to substitute neutron bombs for hydrogen bombs.

Commonly Used Measuring Units

The most familiar measuring unit is the roentgen, abbreviated to *r*. The technical definition need not concern us. For practical purposes, it is enough to consider it a basic unit of radiation measurement. Sometimes, a small unit is needed, and the milliroentgen (abbreviated *mr*) is used—a one-thousandth part of a roentgen.

The daily dose of radioactivity that cosmic rays emit to people at sea level is about $1/10$ of a milliroentgen per day, or about $2\frac{1}{2}$ roentgens in a lifetime.

The roentgen and milliroentgen have certain drawbacks in defining effects on living organisms. Other units have been developed, therefore, which are technically more precise: the *rep*, the *rad*, and the *rem*. For practical civil defense purposes, we can use the terms roentgen, rep, rad, and rem interchangeably when referring to gamma radiation, which is the major problem, but not when we refer to alpha particles, beta particles or neutrons, which are of much less direct importance.

Radioactive Decay

When a radioactive material emits radiation, it changes or "decays" into another material. At times the product of decay is itself radioactive, but eventually the radioactive material decays to a stable element which does not emit any radiation. The time it takes for the original mass to decay to one-half its size is called the "half-life." If a radioactive material has a half-life of one day, only one-half of it will remain at the end of the first day, one-fourth at the end of the second day, one-eighth at the end of the third day, and so forth. Half-lives of radioactive elements vary from one-millionth of a second to thousands of years. Those elements which produce a large amount of radiation in a short period have a short half-life; those which have a long half-life only give off small amounts of radiation each day.

The detonation of a hydrogen bomb produces up to 40 different radioactive elements with differing half-lives. Studies of test explosions have shown that there is no valid half-life figure which can be given for the mixture. However, there is a relationship between elapsed time and decay of radioactivity which is extremely useful for planning purposes. The radioactivity of fallout particles decays to one-tenth of its previous value with each sevenfold increase in elapsed time. Thus, if the radiation level at one hour after detonation (the usual reference point) is 1,000 r per hour, its level at later times will be as follows:

Elapsed time	Radiation rate (r per hour)
1 hour	1,000
7 hours	100
49 hours (2 days)	10
2 weeks	1
14 weeks	0.1

This emphasizes the importance of protection during the first two days. More than half of the radiation given off by fallout in a seven-year period would come in the first seven hours.

Radiation Effects on People

The effects of radiation on people are not completely understood, but there are enough facts available to serve as a general guide. We don't know how radiation damages tissues, but we do know that such damage occurs.

The dosages used in civil defense terminology refer to total body dosages. They are not at all comparable to the partial body dosages used in radiation therapy.

A total body dosage of less than 50 r would probably have little observable effect. With a dose of 50 to 250 r over a period of a week or less, there would be some radiation sickness, but no deaths. As the dose increases beyond 250 r, the deaths increase in frequency, and at about 450 r half of those exposed would die within a month; at about 750 r almost all of those exposed would die. It should be noted that these figures apply to dosages received over a period of a few days. If the radiation is received over a long period, there is time for the body to repair most of the damage. Thus, if radiation were delivered over a period of five years or more, the dose which would kill half of those exposed would be in the order of 5,000 r, about ten times the amount that would kill on acute exposure. This point is important in assessing the long-term dangers from radioactive fallout after a war.

Radiation Shielding

Shielding is the most effective way of protecting against radiation. The extent of the protection depends on the mass of the shielding material. No shielding is ever complete; some rays will always penetrate. However, the number of rays that penetrate can be lowered sufficiently to be harmless. An important concept here is that of the "half-thickness" of a shielding material. A half-thickness is the thickness of a particular material which will reduce the intensity of a particular type of radiation by one half; two half-thicknesses reduce it to one quarter; three to one eighth; four to one sixteenth, and so forth. Fig. 8 is a diagrammatic representation of the half-thickness principle. It should be noted that half-thickness figures for a particular type and energy level of radiation do not apply to other rays.

Thus, the half-thickness figures for gamma rays emanating from fallout do not apply to the higher energy rays emanating from the fireball; (the half-thicknesses for fireball gamma rays are about 50% greater.) However, the fallout gamma rays are the major problem, and at this time the fireball gamma rays are of academic interest because they only involve the area close to the fireball where no survivors are expected unless they have special deep shelters (*see* chapter 51).

Table I lists some of the half-thicknesses of selected materials and also

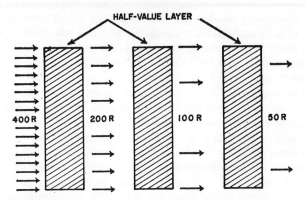

Fig. 8. Representation of the half-value layer thickness.

TABLE I   APPROXIMATE THICKNESS OF MATERIALS NEEDED TO RE-
DUCE THE GAMMA RADIATION FROM FALLOUT

	Reduction to ½	1/100	1/1,000
Steel	0.7 inches	4.5 inches	6.7 inches
Concrete	2.2 inches	14 inches	23 inches
Packed Earth	3.3 inches	21 inches	36 inches
Water	4.8 inches	31 inches	50 inches
Wood	8.8 inches	57 inches	90 inches
Air	200 feet	1,300 feet	2,000 feet

the thicknesses needed to reduce fallout gamma rays by factors of 100 and 1,000.

These values actually depend on the total mass of the shielding material. One hundred pounds of any material provides approximately the same shielding as 100 pounds of any other material for the same area covered. Thus, there is no possibility of developing light, portable shielding materials or "fallout suits."

In civil defense terminology, the reciprocal of the shielding value is called the protection factor. Thus, if a certain thickness of concrete reduces the fallout radiation to 1/100 of its outside level, that thickness of concrete is said to have a protection factor of 100.

Scattering of Radiation

Gamma radiation, like light, is reflected and scattered from certain materials. This reflection is sometimes called "albedo." The ability of surfaces to reflect gamma rays is not directly related to their ability to reflect light. Thus, shiny surfaces do not necessarily reflect more gamma rays than dull surfaces. Surfaces of metal, concrete, and other building materials scatter about 2% of gamma rays around corners. This is not likely to be a problem in most cases, and single right-angle turns are therefore usually considered sufficient for the entrance to fallout shelters.

The atmosphere reflects back to earth about 10% of the gamma rays passing upwards from fallout on the ground. This high reflectivity of the atmosphere—sometimes called "skyshine"—is due to its content of nitrogen. It is responsible for what civil defense publications refer to as the "foxhole effect," a protection factor afforded by a deep foxhole. The earth around the hole effectively blocks out almost all direct radiation from fallout on the ground. The only significant radiation hitting the foxhole's occupant is that reflected from the sky—10% of the amount delivered to someone standing at ground level. Thus, a deep hole in the ground provides a protection factor of ten, even if open at the top. A basement, which is below ground on all sides, has the same protection factor. It seems, then, that the amount of fallout which remains on the roof is negligible in comparison to the fallout on the ground.

Radiation Measuring Instruments

Geiger counters are relatively sensitive radiation measuring devices which indicate intensity of radiation in the low milliroentgen range. The least sensitive Geiger counter registers a maximum of 50 milliroentgens per hour. In a post-attack situation, we would be concerned with radiation levels in the high roentgen range—about 1,000 to 10,000 times the maximum which can be recorded by a Geiger counter. Clearly, then, Geiger counters are not likely to be of much value in a thermonuclear attack. Most of them also have an unfortunate response when exposed to high levels of radiation: instead of registering the maximum, they register zero or close to it. Therefore, Geiger counters could be highly misleading when a radiation level in the roentgen range is present.

Scintillation counters are, in general, even more sensitive than Geiger counters and therefore also of little or no value in a post-attack situation.

Instruments which can measure radiation in the roentgen range are known as radiation detection meters. They are supplied by civil defense authorities to specially trained radiation monitors, and can be purchased by individuals from the manufacturers.

In addition, there are instruments, called dosimeters, which measure the amount of radiation to which a person has already been exposed. Similar instruments are being used in hospitals to measure exposure of radiologists, nurses, and technicians to X-rays.

49 EFFECTS OF HYDROGEN BOMBS

In order to plan protective measures which will be practical and effective, it is necessary to understand the type and extent of the effects produced by weapons which might be employed against us. The following chapters will show how adequate planning and protective measures can markedly reduce the casualties from a hydrogen bomb attack.

The hydrogen bomb produces different effects, depending on whether it detonates on the ground, under water, or in the air. We will first consider the effects of a 20 megaton bomb detonating on the ground. Then, we can consider water and air bursts, and the relationship of bomb size to radius of effect.

The 20 megaton bomb has an explosive capacity equal to 20 million tons of TNT. On detonation at ground level it produces the following effects:

1. Cratering of the soil.
2. Initial nuclear radiation from the fireball.
3. Initial heat radiation from the fireball.
4. Blast effects.
5. Flying debris.
6. Radiation from fallout.

Each of these may be a lethal effect in a wide area, if there is no protection. Table II presents the radius and area of these effects assuming no shelter.

The crater which is formed is about a third of a mile in diameter and several hundred feet deep. The earth which is blown out—several million tons—is made intensely radioactive and becomes dangerous when it descends as fallout.

It should be noted that the term "lethal" in Table II does not mean that every person within the area affected will be killed unless special shelters are available. Since ordinary buildings give some protection, there will be a substantial number of survivors, even in the areas damaged by blast and fire. An estimate by the Department of Defense of the number of survivors after a 20 megaton detonation, *even without special shelters,* is summarized in Table III.

TABLE II POTENTIALLY LETHAL EFFECTS OF A GROUND BURST OF A 20 MEGATON BOMB—NO SHELTER

	Radius		Area
Crater	0.35	miles	
Absolute destruction of an underground shelter	1.0	miles	3 square miles
Initial nuclear radiation	2.5	miles	20 square miles
Blast effects—reinforced concrete building	5	miles	80 square miles
Blast effects—ordinary frame house	10	miles	310 square miles
Flying debris	10	miles	310 square miles
Initial heat radiation	12	miles	450 square miles
Firestorm*	up to 20	miles	
Radioactive fallout	140	miles (oval)	10,000 to 20,000

*This effect would be rare (*see* chapters 33 and 50).

TABLE III ESTIMATES OF PER CENT OF PEOPLE DEAD, INJURED, AND SAFE (INCLUDING MINOR INJURIES) IN POTENTIALLY LETHAL AREAS, WITHOUT SPECIAL SHELTERS (20 MEGATON BOMB)

Distance from ground zero	Damage to buildings	People dead	People injured	People safe
Less than 5 miles	Total	98%	2%	0
5 to 7 miles	Heavy	40%	25%	35%
7 to 11 miles	Moderate	5%	20%	75%
11 to 15 miles	Light	0	10%	90%

Source: Civil Defense-Fallout Shelter Program. Hearings before Subcommittee No. 3: Committee on Armed Services. House of Repr., June-July, 1963, p. 5139.

If the bomb is detonated in the atmosphere, well above ground level, there would be no crater and no appreciable fallout, but there would be blast and heat effects. If the detonation took place high in the stratosphere, the only important effects would be those resulting from the heat radiation.

If a hydrogen bomb were detonated beneath the surface of the water, a large, destructive wave would be formed which could destroy most buildings near the coast. Radioactive fallout would also be a problem. Heat radiation would be minimal and flying debris would be absent.

Bombs of other sizes have effects which are related to the bomb size, but not in a linear fashion. The radius of most effects is proportional to the cube root of the bomb size, and the area of most effects is proportional to the square of the cube root. Some comparisons of different-size bombs are presented in Table IV. It can be seen from this table that the larger

TABLE IV   RELATIONSHIP OF BOMB SIZE TO RADIUS AND AREA OF EFFECTS (IN ARBITRARY UNITS). THIS DOES NOT APPLY TO FIRE.

Bomb size (megatons)	Radius	Area
1	1.00	1.00
2	1.26	1.59
5	1.71	2.92
10	2.15	4.62
20	2.71	7.34
50	3.68	13.48
100	4.64	21.53

bombs are relatively less damaging than the equivalent amount of smaller bombs. Thus, three 20 megaton bombs would be more destructive than one 100 megaton bomb.

The relationships in Table IV do not, however, apply to the fire effects. Because these are complex, they are discussed separately in chapter 50.

The greatest danger from a hydrogen bomb comes from the radioactive fallout. It can be seen from Table II that the area covered by lethal fallout would be 20 to 40 times greater than the area covered by the next greatest potential cause of death. For this reason, the U. S. government has been emphasizing shelters which protect against fallout. We will follow their lead. At the same time, it is important to note that shelters can be built which would give protection against heat and blast well within the area of total destruction of ordinary buildings. Such shelters will be discussed further in chapter 51.

There are some people who dispute the government's position that fallout is the greatest danger from a thermonuclear attack. They contend that firestorms are a greater menace but this is not the case. (*See* chapter 50.)

Radioactive fallout consists of material sucked up from the crater, made radioactive by the neutrons from the bomb, and of particles from the bomb itself. A single explosion produces several million tons of fallout.

The fallout particles are carried for varying distances by the winds in the stratosphere before settling to earth. Each fallout particle may be likened to a tiny X-ray machine, emitting rays in all directions.

Table IV may be used to estimate, from Table II, the effects of a bomb other than 20 megatons. For example, if we wish to estimate the probable lethal blast radius of a 100 megaton bomb (no shelter), knowing that the lethal blast radius of a 20 megaton bomb is ten miles, we use the equation $\dfrac{4.64}{2.71} = \dfrac{X}{10}$. Thus, the lethal blast radius (no shelter) of a 100 megaton bomb is 17 miles.

The fallout particles themselves vary in size, with large ones falling to earth rather rapidly—within 10 to 20 minutes in a circle around ground zero. The area covered by these larger fallout particles is usually about the size of the area involved in blast and fire damage, or slightly larger. Sometimes, this portion of the fallout is called "immediate fallout."

The medium-size fallout particles, about the size of a grain of sand, come to earth over a much larger area. If there are no cross winds, the fallout pattern resembles a fat cigar, with the intensity diminishing as the distance from ground zero increases. However, since the winds in the stratosphere are irregular, the area of fallout is not completely predictable.

The fallout from a 20 megaton bomb extends several hundred miles beyond ground zero, but the potentially lethal area lies usually within 150 miles of ground zero.

The time it takes for this type of fallout to descend ranges from 30 minutes to six hours. This is highly significant. It means that persons who are outside the area of blast and fire damage can expect at least a 30-minute warning time to get into a fallout shelter. This warning comes from the bomb itself and is not dependent on any action of civil defense authorities. The light given off by a hydrogen bomb is far more intense than any other light in human experience and cannot be mistaken for anything else. At a distance of 100 miles from ground zero, the light from a 20 megaton bomb will produce a general illumination about ten times as great as the level present at noon on a bright sunny day. This light lasts almost a full minute, so that it can't be mistaken for lightning (which is much less bright). Everyone in the area subject to fallout will be warned by the bomb-flash of the impending fallout. There will be enough time to get to a suitable shelter, if such shelters are available. In general, most people can walk at least one mile in the interval from bomb-flash to the beginning of fallout, and some will be able to walk several miles.

In other words, the effectiveness of fallout shelters does not depend on any warning devices other than the explosion of the bomb itself.

Fallout radiation loses its intensity rapidly, so that protection, even if only for a short time, could be life-saving. Details of the decay rates of fallout are presented in the preceding chapter.

The smallest fallout particles remain high in the stratosphere and do not descend to earth for several weeks or months. By this time, they have lost most of their radioactivity, and do not present a serious problem in comparison to the other bomb effects.

50 THERMAL EFFECTS OF HYDROGEN BOMBS

The thermal effects of hydrogen bombs include the production of fires, firestorms, burns, and blindness. There has been so much confusion and misinformation about these areas that it seems advisable to devote a chapter to the clarification of these phenomena.

When a hydrogen bomb detonates, it releases a large amount of heat rays, which travel in all directions at the speed of light. If these rays strike inflammable materials at a close enough range, they can start fires; if they strike bare skin at a close enough range, they produce burns, and if they strike the retina of the eye, they may produce a localized burn which in turn results in partial blindness. While these facts are unquestioned, there are some serious misconceptions about the range at which these effects occur, and about their secondary consequences.

Fires

The range at which hydrogen bombs produce ignition of inflammable trash has been studied in early tests of low-yield bombs. Subsequent findings formed the basis on which deductions were made for larger-yield weapons. When it was found that extremely large bombs released a higher percentage of their energy as radiant heat, it was naturally assumed that they could start fires at extremely long ranges. However, later studies showed that the heat energy released by them is considerably *less* effective in causing ignition than that of small bombs. It was once believed that the ignition threshold for newspaper, for instance, for large as well as small bombs was six to eight calories per square centimeter. Recent tests show that for large bombs it is much higher—about 34 calories per square centimeter. Thus, it would take four to five times more heat from a large bomb to start newspapers burning than had previously been thought necessary. An opponent of civil defense testified before a congressional committee that he believed a 30 megaton bomb, detonated at a height of 17 miles, would produce essentially total destruction by fire over a radius of about 42 miles (over 5,500 square miles). However, his deductions were contradicted by a leading government expert who has actually studied fire effects. According to reliable data, a 30 megaton bomb, exploded on a *very clear day,* could start fires only within a five mile radius (or about 78 square miles). If there were some haze or cloud-cover, such a weapon, exploded at that height, would cause no fires at all.

The effectiveness of bombs of all sizes in causing fires is dependent on the clarity of the atmosphere. As a general rule, a haze or cloud cover through which the sun cannot be seen, will block out the thermal rays from a hydrogen bomb so as to prevent fire effects beyond the zone of heavy blast damage. Actually, the average American city has about 120 clear days per year. Thus, there is about one chance in three that any significant fire effects beyond the heavy blast damage area would result from an attack on any particular day. If an enemy attack lasted more than a day, the likelihood is that after the first day, all areas would be protected against thermal effects by the haze in the upper atmosphere, produced by the tiny fallout particles which do not descend to earth for long periods.

Therefore, it can be seen that the ability of hydrogen bombs to cause fires at great distances is much less than has been commonly supposed. On the other hand, extensive fires would be produced within the area of major blast damage (*see* Table II, p. 212).

Firestorms

Firestorms are mass fires that overcome the normal wind structure. A thermal column is produced which draws wind into the firestorm area from all directions, regardless of the initial wind direction. The dangers of firestorms have been exaggerated to an almost incredible degree, and it is important, therefore, to set the record straight.

The conditions which allow a firestorm to develop include a high concentration of combustible material in an area of at least one square mile. At least 20% of the area (some experts say 30%) must be covered by combustible multistoried buildings before a firestorm can develop.* Roads, sidewalks, and yards reduce the coverage of land by inflammable buildings. Single story buildings cannot support a firestorm unless they are packed very closely together. Experts in the Defense Department have conducted studies of American cities and have concluded that there are only six cities in the United States which could develop a firestorm (and only in part of the city) if there were a massive enemy attack.

It must also be pointed out that the nature of the wind pattern in firestorms is such that they do not spread to other areas since all winds blow inwards.

The second misconception about firestorms is that they "deoxygenate" the area. There is clear and conclusive evidence that this not only does not

* Martin, T. L. and Latham, D. C. *Strategy for Survival.* U. of Arizona Press, Tucson, 1963, p. 83.

happen but also cannot happen. There is a slight relative drop in oxygen concentration in the firestorm area, but not enough to cause any difficulty or even to be noticed without special measuring instruments. The fundamental point is that wood requires a much higher oxygen concentration in order to burn than human beings need to breathe and survive indefinitely. Burning wood will stop producing any flame if the oxygen concentration falls below 15%; under that it may smoulder. By contrast, human beings can breathe comfortably for days at oxygen concentrations of 14%. Even at concentrations as low as 10%, people can survive, although they may get headaches. Therefore, if a firestorm area were cut off from the surrounding air so that the oxygen level would fall below 15%, the fire would go out long before the persons in the area would suffer from oxygen lack. This kind of situation occurred in a few tightly closed shelters in Hamburg, where the oxygen content dropped to a point where the candles wouldn't burn. However, the shelter occupants lived to tell of their experience. A firestorm area is not cut off from surrounding air but, as pointed out above, the surrounding air rushes in with great velocity. At ground level in a firestorm area, oxygen levels are quite close to normal; only in the heated column of smoke and flame rising above the firestorm is there any significant decrease in oxygen.

The major hazard in a firestorm area, aside from heat, is not the lack of oxygen but the presence of carbon monoxide. This gas often occurs in lethal concentrations and we have no practical way of removing it. In shelters with a large volume of stored air per person, it is possible to close all openings and breathe the stored air until the firestorm is over. However, this would not be practical in a crowded shelter. In most cases, air could be drawn into the shelter safely, even in a firestorm area, as was done in Hamburg and Hiroshima (*see* below). However, in some cases, bringing in air would kill the occupants. Protection could be provided by supplying a source of oxygen and a means of removing carbon dioxide. It should be emphasized again that the provision of oxygen is not due to deoxygenation of the area but to the danger of carbon monoxide; also, it is easier and cheaper to seal a shelter and provide oxygen than it is to try and filter out or absorb the carbon monoxide. The cost of providing oxygen is not excessive—about $15.00 to $20.00 per person for the duration of the longest firestorm. Materials to provide this protection are already commercially available.

The third misconception about firestorms is that all persons in a firestorm area will die unless they can take refuge in hermetically sealed, insulated, air-conditioned shelters with a self-contained oxygen supply.

This assumption has been disproved by the experiences in the Hiroshima and Hamburg firestorms.

After the atom bombing of Hiroshima, there was a firestorm with a radius of about 1.2 miles (area approximately 4.5 miles). Persons in the traditional Japanese buildings perished, but most of those in American-style concrete buildings survived. This is illustrated diagrammatically in Fig. 9. These survivors were inside the firestorm, and their buildings surrounded by flames.

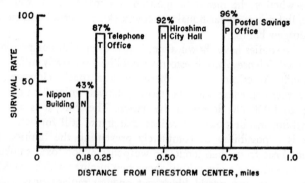

Fig. 9. Survival in American-style buildings in Hiroshima.

In Hamburg, most of those in the firestorm area survived. A British analysis of the firestorm, made after the war, is of considerable interest. It noted the following:

Total population of Hamburg 1,500,000
Population in area raided and heavily damaged 470,000
Population within the firestorm area 280,000
Number killed in firestorm 40,000

Thus, the number of survivors amounted to 86% of those actually inside the firestorm area, 93% of those in the raided and damaged area, and 97% of the total population of the city.

An analysis of the survival rate by type of shelter is also interesting. Of the 280,000 people inside the firestorm, 53,000 were in bunkers and good shelters; their survival rate was approximately 100%. An additional 227,000 people were in less satisfactory basement shelters; of these, 40,000 died, and 187,000, or more than 82%, survived.

Let us state again that most of the survivors in the Hiroshima and Hamburg firestorms did not have special air-conditioned shelters or indeed anything more elaborate than those which would be available to

Americans under the government's present program. There is every reason to believe, then, that most Americans would also survive in a firestorm area. The fact that a firestorm might be started by a hydrogen bomb rather than by an atom bomb, or by thermite bombs, is of little or no importance. The heat, intensity, and duration of a firestorm do not depend on the method of ignition but on the type, concentration, and arrangement of the fuel. If adequate fuel lies in the path of a firestorm and if the early fires are not extinguished, the intensity of the storm will be approximately the same whether the means of ignition is a match, a thermite bomb, a cigarette, lightning, an earthquake, a cow kicking over a kerosene lantern, or a hydrogen bomb.

What the studies have shown, then, is that even with our present facilities and civil defense plans, firestorms would be a relatively minor cause of death among Americans after a thermonuclear attack. However, in discussing a thermonuclear war, the term "relatively minor" might still involve up to 1,000,000 deaths in the nation. Therefore, it is advisable to do everything in our power to reduce that figure still further.

There is a possibility of completely preventing the ignition of fires by radiant heat from thermonuclear weapons: a non-toxic smoke screen could be spread over a city within about two minutes which would persist for many hours, and would block out enough radiant heat to prevent burns or fires. The cost would be quite low—less than 25 cents for each person protected. There are indications that the government is considering this measure, but no concrete steps have as yet been taken.

On the other hand, there are no known methods of preventing fires and firestorms in the area of severe blast damage. The broken gas mains and electric lines here would probably be enough to start fires even if radiant heat from the fireball could be blocked out. The chances of survival in this area, nevertheless, would be substantial if one employed the type of protection currently being suggested by the U. S. government. However, the chances of survival could be increased by the use of fireproof, blast-resistant shelters. The cost of these would be about $200 per person for the family-sized unit, and less for community or neighborhood shelters.

Burns

Radiant heat from the fireball can produce burns on exposed skin at considerable ranges on a clear day. However, clothing, buildings, and the curvature of the earth generally block out enough of the radiant heat to prevent burns. Most people are fully clothed most of the time; in addition, burns occur only on the side of the body that faces the fireball.

Thus, even a completely naked person would incur burns of no more than 50% of his body. Most burns would occur on the face and on women's legs. It is probable that there would be some deaths from burns produced by radiant heat outside the zone of heavy damage, and there would most likely be many non-fatal burns. The smoke screen mentioned above could prevent almost all of these burns; personal preventive measures such as wearing appropriate clothing and remaining indoors would also help.

Blindness

The subject of blindness as a result of looking at the fireball has also been greatly exaggerated and confused. If anyone is looking in the direction of the fireball at the instant of detonation, blindness could ensue. The first pulse of radiant heat waves is emitted so rapidly that the waves would damage the retina even before the blink reflex can operate. If the observer were standing fairly close to the fireball, his entire retina would be burned, causing blindness. At great distances from the fireball, some retinal damage could theoretically still be produced. As the distance increases, the intensity of heat radiation falls off. However, the lens of the eye concentrates the rays (just as a magnifying glass can concentrate the sun's rays), and this could produce a localized burn of the retina. The area of the retina that is burned would be in proportion to the size of the image cast on the retina. At considerable distances, therefore, the major possible damage would be a tiny blind spot on the retina, not total blindness, even on a very clear day; haze or cloudiness would greatly reduce the range of retinal damage.

It must be emphasized that these effects would only occur in persons who happened to be looking directly at the fireball at the instant of detonation, others would not be affected. There has been some discussion among opponents of civil defense of a so-called "uncontrollable reflex" which would force everyone to look at the fireball and thus become blind. This is completely at variance with basic physiologic facts. Persons walking out of their homes in the morning to a bright sunny street do not have an "uncontrollable reflex" forcing them to look at the sun; most people tend to look away from the bright sun. (The reader can test this himself on a sunny day.)

Secondly, even if we were to assume, for the sake of argument, that someone did have some unusual reflex forcing him to look at the fireball, he still would not be blinded. The blink reflex, which is extremely rapid, would close his eyes long before the head and neck could be twisted to look at the light.

The danger of blindness, exaggerated as it is, does, however, exist. It can be minimized both by government action (use of smoke screens) and by individual protective methods. Some of the latter include remaining in a building when warned of an attack, covering the head and face, looking downward while walking, and driving with one eye covered.

Temporary Flash Blindness

Temporary flash blindness is likely to cause more problems than retinal burns. In order to develop temporary flash blindness, one need not be looking directly at the fireball. The general intense light could cause excessive bleaching of the visual purple of the retina, so that hours or even a day or two might be needed for recovery. Temporary flash blindness is likely to occur in persons who are outdoors or near a window within 30 miles of ground zero of a 20 megaton detonation. These persons would need help in getting to a shelter. They should be reassured and told their blindness is only temporary.

There are several protective measures which can be taken. In most cases, the blink reflex would prevent flash blindness from the large bombs which release light more slowly than the small ones. Citizens should be instructed to keep both eyes tightly closed and covered with their hands for a full two minutes after the first blink. If there has been any warning of an impending attack, either from government sources or from the light flashes of bombs, bursting more than 100 miles away a few seconds earlier, those who can do so should lie down, covering their eyes with their hands. Citizens who are walking or driving to a shelter should proceed with only one eye open, and with the other one closed and protected by their hands or by some opaque material put over an eyeglass lens. Then, if temporary flash blindness hits one eye, the other can be used to get to the shelter.

As we have seen, the dangers of fire, firestorm, burns, and blindness have been exaggerated. There may be some who will disagree with the position taken in this chapter, but let them note that the critical statements of fact are supported by authoritative studies.

The following conclusions, therefore, seem warranted:

1. The range at which hydrogen bombs would cause serious fires would be approximately equal to the range of blast damage, i.e., about ten miles for a 20 megaton bomb.

2. Bombs larger than 20 megatons would be relatively *less* effective in starting fires.

3. There are probably only six cities in the United States which have areas that could be seriously involved in a firestorm.

4. The haze and cloud cover which lie over most cities would reduce the number of cities likely to be involved in a firestorm to less than six.

5. Most persons could survive a firestorm in large concrete and steel buildings, or in properly designed shelters.

6. Firestorms do not and cannot reduce the available oxygen to a level dangerous to people.

7. The causes of death in firestorms are heat and carbon monoxide, not lack of oxygen.

8. The danger of permanent blindness from looking at the fireball would be quite small if people understood basic civil defense protective measures.

9. The thermal effects of a hydrogen bomb are far less serious than the effects of radioactive fallout.

51 PROTECTION AGAINST FALLOUT RADIATION

Since fallout radiation is the most dangerous effect of a hydrogen bomb detonation, protection against such radiation is the most important single action. There are three basic factors which provide protection: time, distance, and shielding.

The effect of time is based on the rapid decay of radioactivity from fallout. For every sevenfold increase in elapsed time, there is a tenfold decrease in radiation intensity (chapter 49). Therefore, if one is protected against radiation for 49 hours (two days), the radiation levels will be only 1/100 of the levels at one hour after detonation. For many people, protection for two days would be sufficient. In some areas of high radiation intensity, protection may be needed for two weeks. Upon emerging from a shelter after two weeks (7 x 7 x 7 hours) the outside radiation levels would be only 1/1,000 of those at one hour after detonation.

The protection afforded by time may also be used to "stretch out" shelter facilities. For the first seven hours, maximum protection would be needed. People could be crowded into the safest shelter area in a large building. After seven hours, when the radiation intensity is down to 10% of its one-hour level, it would be safe to move some of the people into less protected parts of the building. After 48 hours, with the level down to 1%, people could safely use most areas of most large buildings.

Distance is a protective factor which applies to certain types of large buildings. For example, the lower and upper floors in skyscrapers are close to the radioactive fallout particles and do not give much protection. However, the middle floors are far enough away to have a relatively high protection factor. This presumes that there are no balconies or exterior ornaments around the middle floors on which fallout might collect. The geometry of the protective effect of distance may often be complex, since a particular building's protection factor may be influenced by buildings around it.

In some cases, such as Navy vessels and installations, the protective effect of distance is obtained from a washing technique. Water is hosed or sprayed over contaminated surfaces to wash the radioactive particles away. It should be noted that water in no way reduces radioactivity. It merely moves the radioactive particles from a vulnerable area to one where they can do less harm.

Shielding is the interposition of a mass of material between the source of radioactivity and the persons to be protected. The shield absorbs most of the radiation, so that only a small proportion gets through. Special shielding against alpha and beta particles is unnecessary. However, gamma rays are so penetrating that shielding is needed. In theory, any material could be used as a shield—if it were thick enough. One pound of any material provides about the same degree of shielding as one pound of any other material. However, most materials are impractical as shields for one reason or another. Lead, steel, and wood are impractical because of their high cost per pound. (A family fallout shelter depending on lead for its shielding would cost about $25,000.) On the other hand, steel and wood are practical for use as structural supports to hold up cheaper shielding material. The most practical shielding materials are earth, rock, and concrete. Earth and crushed rock weigh about 100 pounds per cubic foot, and concrete about 150 pounds.

Of the several types of shelters that are practical, let us first consider the community shelter. Such a shelter may be located in a soundly constructed large building. Basements are the most common shelter areas, although the middle floors of skyscrapers are also suitable. Some areas need no modifications at all; others may need slight alterations. The federal government has marked and stocked many community shelters, but it is important to remember that these are fallout shelters, and no claim has been made that they will provide protection against blast or fire.

Among community shelters that may be constructed, the most efficient and economical are those that are excavated in rock. They provide protection against blast and fire, as well as fallout. There are many such shelters in Sweden but relatively few in the United States. They are practical only if certain types of rock formation are present.

There are several types of family shelters that have been described in civil defense publications. One type is made of a corrugated steel pipe covered with three to five feet of earth. This would provide a radiation protection factor of 5,000 to 50,000, plus protection against a firestorm overhead and against blast. Occupants of such a shelter could expect to survive a 20 megaton detonation only two to three miles away. These shelters can be built at a cost only slightly greater than the basement-room shelter, if built to order by a steel fabricator. Accordingly, it is suggested that anyone contemplating the building of a family shelter investigate the corrugated steel shelter.

There are also ready-made shelters which have been extensively advertised. Some are good and some are not; all of them are excessively expensive.

There are some other basic principles that concern shelters which should be considered.

Under certain situations, protection factors multiply. It has been pointed out (chapter 48) that a deep basement with all four walls below ground level has a protection factor of ten (a foxhole effect). If a shelter with an additional protection factor of ten is built in that basement, the total protection inside the shelter is 10 x 10 or 100. This is the basis of the home fallout shelter recommended by the Office of Civil Defense. This principle of multiplying protection factors may be used to provide important extra protection within some shelters. After a thermonuclear attack, some people may not be able to get to a good shelter and may have to take refuge in a building with a protection factor of only 25 or 50. It may be possible, though, to build in a few minutes a small cubicle consisting of a table with books or cartons piled on top and around the sides. While this would only give a protection factor of about three or four, it would, *multiplied* by the basic protection factor of the building, give a reasonably adequate degree of protection for the critical first seven hours.

The multiplication of protection factors, however, only applies where there are no gaps or weak points in the defensive shield. Just as a chain is as strong as its weakest link, a shelter is as good as its weakest side (or roof). Accordingly, care must be taken to see that doors and openings (including ducts) are staggered and not in a direct line; this will prevent rays from coming directly into the shelter.

The space allotted to each person is ten square feet, or about 70 cubic feet in above-ground shelters and in below-ground shelters which are ventilated. In basement shelters which are not ventilated, the space allotted is 500 cubic feet per person.

Federal authorities state that in most areas of the nation, filtration of incoming air would not be necessary. However, suitable filters and blowers are commercially available at a moderate cost for those who wish to purchase them.*

Packaged food is not injured by radioactive fallout. The fallout particles can be brushed or wiped off; the food would then be safe to eat. Some types of unpackaged food may be safe to eat even if stored in containers contaminated by fallout, provided it is practical to wash or peel the food. This should be done according to directions of the civil defense authorities.

* Garb, S. Providing Safe Ventilation. *N. Y. State J. of Med.,* 60: 3292, 1960; also *Missouri Medicine, 59:* 780, 1962.

Water from deep wells would be free of any radioactive contamination, while surface water is likely to be unsafe for drinking for some time. However, radioactive material dissolved or suspended in water can be removed efficiently by several processes. One is the use of ion exchange resins (as in water softeners), another is distillation, and still another is filtration through a column of uncontaminated earth. *To boil water does not remove or reduce its radioactivity.*

It is advisable for each family to have a survival plan. This plan should include knowing the location of several fallout shelters, so that if the first-choice shelter is already filled on arrival, the family could proceed in a rapid, orderly way to another shelter. Some families might be separated at the time of an attack, and a family plan should emphasize survival of all members of the family, rather than keeping them together as a unit. It is better, even for a child, to be separated from his parents for two or more days than it is to subject it to even 30 minutes of shelterless exposure shortly after the detonation of a hydrogen bomb. A family plan should also include several prearranged meeting points and times for the period when it is safe again to leave the shelters.

In most cases, local civil defense directors will be happy to help families develop their survival plans. However, this must be done well *before* any international crisis. During a crisis, civil defense directors are unable to give much attention to the problems of individual families.

It is possible that if a sudden international crisis makes an attack seem imminent, many people will not have any shelters to go to. There are, however, makeshift shelters which can be constructed by neighborhood groups within 24 hours.

Questions have been raised about the value of fallout shelters to city dwellers. Careful studies by competent officials have shown that they would be extremely valuable: fully half the lives which might be saved by fallout shelters would be those of city dwellers.*

The long-term effects of fallout radiation would pose serious problems to the survivors of an attack. Despite the fact that this area has been a source of extensive misinformation and confusion, these problems can be solved by intelligent analysis and planning. Considerable attention has been given in the newspapers to comparatively minor long-term effects, while the more serious ones have been largely ignored. The incidence of birth deformities would increase slightly—from the present level of 4% to 5% of total births. The effects on bird and insect life would not serious-

* Civil Defense; Fallout Shelter Program. Hearings Before Subcommittee No.3. Committee on Armed Services, House of Repr., June-July 1963, p. 5121.

ly affect man. There have been statements that the fallout radiation would kill all the birds but spare the insects, with the result that the insects, freed of nature's control, would multiply rapidly and destroy all crops. Actually, there are relatively few insectivorous birds; insects are kept in check by other predatory insects, by spiders, and by chemical insecticides. Even if all birds were killed, our agriculture would not be seriously hampered. Furthermore, since birds are exceedingly mobile, birds from other areas would fly in within a year or two, and their progeny would fill the void.

As mentioned before, the major problem of long-term effects of fallout radiation has received little public attention. Reliable and informed scientists have calculated that a major attack, within the capability of a potential enemy (7,000 megatons), would—in the absence of proper protective measures—produce enough strontium-90 to kill 50% of all children through leukemia and bone cancer.* This would apply not only to children surviving the attack but also to those born for about five or ten years after. Fortunately, there are ways of reducing this toll to a level of less than 5%, once the problem and its solutions are generally recognized. Unfortunately, however, our research efforts in cancer and leukemia are receiving only a fraction of the support which they deserve.

* *Shielding Symposium Proceedings.* U. S. Naval Radiological Defense Laboratory, Washington, D. C., 1960, p. 134.

52 SPECIAL MEDICAL AND NURSING CIVIL DEFENSE PROBLEMS

In planning their civil defense roles, the doctor and nurse must not only provide for the survival of themselves and their families, but must also be prepared to render practical assistance to other survivors. The first principle to keep firmly in mind is that a dead or dying doctor or nurse is of no value to other survivors. There is a great danger that doctors and nurses who survive the initial blast may, in their eagerness to help other survivors, lose their own lives needlessly.

For every doctor or nurse who dies we may estimate that about 200 short-term survivors, who might have been saved by appropriate care in the six weeks following an attack, will also die. Unfortunately, some of the original plans for the use of doctors and nurses in a thermonuclear attack included some basic defects which could have caused the needless deaths of all involved. Thus, it is vital to understand the defects in such plans and to revise them accordingly.

At one time, there were plans to transport doctors and nurses into the impact area to render assistance to people with mechanical injuries from blast and flying objects. Let us consider this in the light of what we now know about the hydrogen bomb's effects. A 20 megaton bomb will produce mechanical injuries from blast, collapsing houses, and flying objects over a radius of 10 miles (314 square miles). For a few minutes after the blast, there will be no fallout; then, after a variable interval—depending on several factors—fallout will occur. We cannot predict exactly when the fallout will descend in this area, but it should begin within 30 minutes. This so-called immediate fallout is far more intense than the distant fallout which will extend over tens of thousands of square miles. Also, it covers the entire blast-damage area, regardless of wind direction. At H hour $+ 1$, the fallout radiation level in the blast damage area would be about 5,000 r per hour. Exposure for *six minutes* or less would be lethal to persons not in shelters. Doctors and nurses going into such an area soon after an attack would certainly perish. Furthermore, their deaths would be useless, since any patients exposed in that area would also have received a lethal dose of radiation in these few minutes.

Therefore, it is recommended that doctors, nurses, and other persons avoid going into any blast-damage area for at least two days after an attack, and preferably for at least two weeks. Patients in the blast-damage area probably cannot be saved by anyone from other areas during the first two days. This does not mean, however, that they must be abandoned to die. Adequate civil defense preparations and training of the population could save the lives of many who are injured by blast. The major requirements are that there be enough community shelters in the area, and that most of the population learn the basic first-aid measures. One basic first-aid principle will have to be changed, however. The principle of "splint them where they lie" is not applicable to a hydrogen bomb blast. The immediate fallout may come down within 10 or 20 minutes, too short an interval for splinting and transporting casualties. Furthermore, the radiation intensity at 10 or 20 minutes after H hour may be over 20,000 r per hour, so that a *two-minute* exposure would be lethal. A first-aid worker, busy splinting a casualty would not have enough time to get to a shelter himself in such a situation. There is only one apparent solution to this problem: the injured must be carried or dragged to the nearest shelter at once by the nearest companions, *without* splinting or first aid. Once inside the shelter, first-aid measures may be instituted. This is certainly a severe solution and undoubtedly the movement of unsplinted fracture patients to shelters will, in many instances, precipitate shock and cause other fatal complications. Nevertheless, this procedure offers a reasonable chance of survival to the fracture patient who can be moved to a shelter within ten minutes. The alternate procedure, splinting in place before movement to shelter, would result in close to 100% deaths of fracture patients from fallout, as well as the unnecessary deaths of an equivalent number of first-aid personnel.

The training of the entire population in basic first-aid measures for use inside the shelter would certainly be of major value. In addition, there should be people with more advanced first-aid training who can assume greater responsibility, particularly since there will not be nearly enough doctors and nurses to go around.

Clearly, each doctor and nurse will be faced with an impossible workload compared to peacetime standards. In many cases, a single physician or nurse may have to care for 200 seriously ill patients with no other professional help. In such circumstances, it will be necessary to form a plan designed to save as many lives as possible. The first points to consider are the estimated types and proportions of casualties. These are discussed below as percentages of the total incapacitated—not as percentages of the total population. Since some persons will suffer more than one type of injury, the total percentage will be greater than 100. It should also be noted that these percentages are based on the areas involved in different effects of the hydrogen bomb. There would be marked variations from place to place and the estimates are for the nation as a whole, based on our present civil defense accomplishments. Obviously, with more effective civil defense the proportions would change.

Types of Injuries

1. Killed outright—approximately 10% of total casualties.

2. Multiple injuries in blast damage zone which would be fatal even with the best treatment—10%. There is no reasonable likelihood that most persons in this group could even receive the benefit of narcotic drugs to ease their last moments.

3. Fractures and lacerations in blast damage zone not able to receive professional care because doctors and nurses are not in the shelter—5%.

This substantial group of patients will depend for survival on the training and ability of laymen who are in the same shelter. Therefore, it is recommended that a large proportion of the population be trained in advanced first-aid techniques, so that they can give the most effective care possible to these injured. We have a nucleus in former military medical aid men, boy scouts, and others. Volunteers from these groups could be taught enough advanced first aid to save many lives.

4. Fractures and lacerations in blast zone able to receive initial professional care because a doctor or nurse happens to be in the shelter—less than 1%. These cases will have a reasonably good chance of survival even without additional planning.

5. Lacerations from broken glass in areas 10 to 50 miles from ground zero—5%. These victims are likely to swamp existing hospitals, unless trained and taught to take a better course. They will have a grace period of 30 to 90 minutes before fallout descends. If they go to hospitals unprepared to shelter them from fallout, they will probably die of fallout radiation. A better solution would be to have these victims go to shelters where advanced first-aid workers can stop bleeding with pressure bandages and give other life-saving care. After a period of two days to two weeks, it may be possible to get professional surgical help to repair the worst cases.

6. Burn cases with chance for survival—20%. Most of these will be flash burns, sustained at distances up to 25 miles from ground zero. The usual peacetime treatment for burns which takes so much professional care—much more than major surgery—would not be possible.

Here, too, the training of advanced first-aid workers in emergency treatment of burns, including the oral administration of the appropriate mixture of salt and bicarbonate of soda, would save many lives.

7. Radiation sickness—80%. Radiation sickness is likely to be the major effect of a thermonuclear attack. It would be seen all through the nation, except in persons who get to a good shelter promptly, and stay there for the proper length of time. Radiation sickness cases would begin soon after the attack and increase in frequency up to about two weeks after the last weapon is detonated. The details of diagnosis and treatment are described in many excellent publications and need not be repeated here. However, it is appropriate to point out that there are no specific anti-radiation drugs available. The major therapeutic modality will be good general nursing care. This is a time-consuming job. A single doctor or nurse may have to be responsible for hundreds of these patients. In such a situation, it is obviously impossible for a doctor or nurse to provide the care personally. Instead, they will have to recruit, train, and direct others in the basic techniques of caring for the sick. Any training which can be done before the emergency will be of great value in saving lives.

An adequate shelter program would markedly reduce the number of cases of radiation sickness. However, even with a good shelter program, there would probably still be a substantial number of them. Some people may delay in getting to shelters, others may leave the shelter too early, and in some cases, shelters with minimum protective shielding may reduce the radiation dosage below the lethal level, but not below the level producing sickness.

8. Secondary epidemics—10% to 90%. Secondary epidemics have frequently accompanied wars and killed more people than weapons. After an attack, there will be multiple dangers from epidemics, even if the attacker does not use agents of biological warfare. The usual epidemic diseases—typhoid, for instance—already have endemic foci within this country. Bubonic plague exists in some of the wild rodents (sylvatic plague). Generally speaking, though, epidemic diseases are kept under control by our excellent sanitary facilities. After a thermonuclear attack, many of these facilities would be destroyed. Unless stringent action is taken, these diseases could sweep the nation. First, it will be necessary to teach the public the need for strict sanitation. Secondly, regulations for purifying water and disposing of excreta will have to be established and rigidly enforced for an indefinite period after an attack. Clearly, any meas-

ures which could be taken in peacetime would help to make the problem more manageable.

It would be a great help if everyone maintained their immunity to smallpox and tetanus by periodic boosters. Special risk groups should also be immunized against typhoid and typhus.

Another problem is that under the stress and crowding of post-attack living, microorganisms which have not usually been dangerous will overwhelm the body defenses of some persons, become more virulent, and start epidemics. An effective defense would be the maintenance of good general health. Nutrition should be adequate—and we have the surplus food to make it so.

In addition, efforts should be made to see that everyone has adequate rest in the post-attack phase. Some volunteers may try to work too hard and too long. Although their intentions are good, they may unwittingly start or help spread an epidemic of respiratory disease by lowering their own resistance. Doctors, nurses, and other responsible, trained persons should insist that no one go without adequate rest. This applies also to the doctors and nurses themselves.

Stockpiling Medical Supplies

The medical and nursing professions should participate more actively in the planning for stockpiles of medical and surgical supplies for emergency use. In some categories, we now have a large stockpile, but in others, our stockpiles appear to be inadequate.

It may be helpful to discuss a few of the items which are, or should be, stockpiled. The list of supplies is by no means inclusive, but is merely a set of examples. It is hoped that more extensive participation by the medical and nursing professions will result in identifying and correcting other areas of imbalance.

Narcotics. Our stockpile of morphine, according to newspaper reports, is adequate. One wonders, though, how the morphine is going to get from the warehouses to the patients in time to do any good. Morphine would be needed within minutes to hours of an attack, and would do little good two or three days later. Furthermore, morphine is of no value and may even be contraindicated in radiation sickness and other late effects of a hydrogen bomb attack.

Anti-emetics. The drugs which have anti-emetic actions could be of tremendous value in managing radiation sickness. A characteristic feature of radiation sickness is vomiting. If the total radiation dose is administered within a short time, the vomiting may last for a few hours only. However, if the radiation is absorbed over a period of days, which could be the case with many victims after an attack, the vomiting tendency could also last for days. Vomiting is not only uncomfortable—it can, and has been, fatal. We are now so accustomed to the availability of parenteral fluids that we sometimes tend to forget how serious persistent vomiting can be in their absence. It is generally considered that a person who receives 200 r of radiation will survive although he will vomit, and have other symptoms. However, this is based on the availability of our peacetime therapeutic measures. After a thermonuclear attack, when parenteral fluids are not available, a person who receives 200 r of radiation and vomits for a day or two may die of the added effects of dehydration and electrolyte imbalance. The anti-emetic drugs have been proven effective against the vomiting induced by radiation. They can be given orally or by injection, and are relatively inexpensive, compact, easy to store, and have a long storage life. They also have tranquillizing effects. The best are probably the chlorpromazine derivatives. If one had a group of several hundred patients with radiation sickness, beginning to vomit, it would be impossible to give them parenteral fluids, even if such fluids were available. However, the anti-emetic drugs could stop most of the vomiting and save the lives of most of the patients. Accordingly, it is recommended that these drugs be stockpiled in large quantities. Apparently, they are not being stockpiled as yet.

Antibiotics. The need for stockpiling antibiotics seems obvious. Apparently, some stockpiling is being done but there is reason to believe that the amount being stocked is only a small proportion of the probable need.

Vaccines. Some stockpiling of vaccines is taking place, but apparently it, too, is quite inadequate.

Surgical instruments. This has been discussed in chapter 15.

Blood transfusion apparatus. The development of plastic containers for blood has simplified the problem of stockpiling. The limited life of bank blood is still the major obstacle to the storage of large amounts of whole blood. However, vigorous research in this area might provide a solution. In the meantime, blood transfusion apparatus could be stored in large amounts, using minimum space and at relatively low cost. After an emergency, the uninjured could then provide fresh blood for their injured and sick fellow patients. To be sure, this would only be of limited benefit since there wouldn't be enough doctors, nurses, or technologists to draw, match and administer all the blood needed. Nevertheless, it could be used to save many lives. But we are not aware of any substantial stockpiling of this type of apparatus as yet.

Portable hospitals. There is a substantial number of portable hospitals stored on the periphery of target areas. This stockpiling seems to be reasonably effective. However, some calculations suggest that the number of hospitals stored is only a fraction of the number which would be needed. Furthermore, there seem to be some serious omissions in the planning. A 200-bed hospital would require the services of more than 200 helpers. The total number of persons involved would require substantial toilet facilities, especially since diarrhea is a symptom of one stage of radiation sickness, and because the need to avoid secondary epidemics will be great. Existing plans call for establishing emergency hospitals in schools, churches, armories, etc. Presumably, the existing toilet facilities in these buildings are to be used. However, such toilets can only work if their water pipes are intact and if there is electric power available at the pumping station. (The portable gasoline generators used with portable hospitals would not be adequate.) Since any major attack would probably put these services out of commission for a long period of time, a shortage of toilet facilities could cripple the operation of emergency hospitals and spread epidemics. Accordingly, it seems advisable to include an adequate number of portable, collapsible field toilets with each emergency hospital.

Use of Professional Personnel other than Physicians

In the event of a thermonuclear attack, the number of physicians available will be far too small to give even reasonably adequate care to the injured and sick. Accordingly, plans have been developed to utilize other professional groups with some medical or paramedical background in place of physicians. The American Medical Association, on April 15, 1959, presented a plan for emergency medical care, including usage of other professional groups. Unfortunately, this plan seems not to be widely known among the groups who will be responsible for implementing it. It is suggested that each physician obtain a copy of this and any subsequent reports and familiarize himself with it. In addition, the medical profession in each area should provide preparation and training to health personnel other than physicians, so that they may perform their assigned tasks effectively. The professions discussed in the AMA report include: veterinarians, dentists, nurses, technicians, technologists, therapists, optometrists, podiatrists, pharmacists, social workers, psychologists, dieticians, and ambulance drivers.

It may be helpful to consider some of the additional functions recommended for nurses. These include:

1. First aid, including (but not limited to) artificial respiration, emergency treatment of open chest wounds, relief of pain, treatment of shock, and preparation of casualties for movement.

2. Maintenance of patent airway, including intratracheal catheterization and emergency tracheotomy.

3. Control of hemorrhage.

4. Cleansing and treatment of wounds.

5. Bandaging and splinting.

6. Management of psychologically disturbed persons.

7. Management of all normal deliveries.

8. Operation of treatment and aid stations.

Other functions are also listed in the AMA report, and it is likely that subsequent revisions will include additional responsibilities, such as management of burn cases.

It should be noted that the emergency functions assigned to these other professional groups include major segments of current medical and surgical practice. They should not be confused with ordinary first-aid or self-help training programs.

The subjects discussed in this chapter should demonstrate clearly the need for greater participation of physicians, nurses, and other professional personnel in civil defense planning. If these groups do not participate more actively in such planning, we can hardly expect to avoid serious errors and deficiencies in the program.

Bibliography

Air Force Manual: Medical Planning for Disaster Casualty Control. AFM 160-37, Washington, D. C., 1962.

Altman, J. W. et al. *Psychological and Social Adjustment in a Simulated Shelter.* Office of Civil Defense, Superintendent of Documents, Washington, D. C., 1961.

American Medical Association Report on National Emergency Medical Care. Chicago, 1959.

Chandler, C. C. *A Study of Mass Fires and Conflagrations.* U. S. Forest Service, Pacific Southwest Forest and Range Experiment Station, Berkeley, California, 1963.

Civil Defense: Fallout Shelter Program. Hearings Before Subcommittee #3. Committee on Armed Services, House of Representatives, May, June, July, 1963; Washington, D. C.

Civil Defense, 1962. Hearings Before a Subcommittee of the Committee on Government Operations, House of Representatives, Feb. 1962, Washington, D. C.

Conrow, A. C. and White, J. A. New Hospital Digs in for Fall-Out Safety. *Modern Hospital,* 100:112, March 1963.

Effects of Biological Warfare Agents for Use in Readiness Planning. Emergency Manual Guide, Department of Health, Education, and Welfare, Washington, D. C., 1959.

Effects of Chemical Warfare Agents for Use in Readiness Planning. Emergency Manual Guide, Department of Health, Education, and Welfare, Washington, D. C., 1959.

Garb, S., Basic Dietary Supplies and Equipment for Shelters, *N. Y. State J. of Med.,* 60:3666, 1960, and *Missouri Medicine,* 60:46, 1963.

Garb, S. Basic Principles of Protection from Hydrogen Bombs. *N. Y. State J. of Med.,* 60:2897, 1960 and *Missouri Medicine,* 59:422, 1962.

Garb, S. Civil Defense Against Agents of Chemical and Biological Warfare. *Missouri Medicine,* 60:152, 1963.

Garb, S. Civil Defense Planning for Schools. *Missouri Medicine,* 60:257, 1963.

Garb, S., and Keats, T. Family, Neighborhood and Community Shelters. *Missouri Medicine,* 59:348, 1962.

Garb, S. Long Term Survival After a Thermonuclear War. *Missouri Medicine,* 60:446, 1963.

Garb, S. Providing Safe Ventilation, *N. Y. State J. of Med.,* 60:3292, 1960, and *Missouri Medicine,* 59:780, 1962.

Garb, S. Shelters in Rock. *Missouri Medicine,* 59:1088, 1962.

Garb, S. Special Civil Defense Problems of Rural Areas. *Missouri Medicine,* 60:860, 1963.

Garb, S. Special Medical and Nursing Civil Defense Problems. *Missouri Medicine*, 61:111, 1964.

Garb, S. The Types of Shelters Useful for Families. *Missouri Medicine*, 59: 874, 1962.

Glass, A. J. Psychological Problems in Nuclear Warfare. *Am J. of Nursing*, 57:1428, 1957.

Glasstone, S. *The Effects of Nuclear Weapons.* U. S. Government Printing Office, Washington, D. C., 1962.

Goldstein, J. D. and Werley, H. H. Care of Casualties Caused by Nuclear Weapons. *Am. J. of Nursing*, 56:1576, 1956.

Krayhill, H. F. Radiological Hazards in Processed Foods Resulting From Nuclear Warfare. *Food Technology*, 16:13, 1962.

Lewis, K. H. Biological Warfare Hazards in Processed Foods. *Food Technology*, 16:17, 1962.

Martin, T. L. and Latham, D. C. *Strategy for Survival.* U. of Arizona Press, Tucson, 1963.

Ostrom, T. R. *Radiological Decontamination of Food and Water in Nuclear War.* Walter Reed Army Institute of Research, Washington, D. C., 1960.

Parnell, F. L. The Capabilities of Chemical, Biological and Radiological Warfare Agents. *Food Technology*, 16:15, 1962.

Personnel Shelters and Protective Construction. Navdocks, P-81, Department of the Navy, Washington, D. C., Sept. 1961.

Russell, P. W. and Kimbrel, L. G. Estimates of the Kill Probability in Target Area Family Shelters, *J. A. M. A.,* 180:25, 1962.

Shielding Symposium Proceedings. U. S. Naval Radiological Defense Laboratory, Washington, D. C., 1960.

INDEX

A particular disaster is indexed only when it is referred to in the text. Lists of disasters, in chronological order, are included in the chapters of section III: Major Types of Disasters.